LEARNING DISABILITIES INFORMATION FOR TEENS THIRD EDITION

LEARNING DISABILITIES INFORMATION FOR TEENS THIRD EDITION

Health Tips about Academic Skills Disorders and Other Disabilities
That Affect Learning

Including Information about Common Signs of Learning Disabilities, School
Issues, Career Options, Employment Support, and Learning to Live with a
Learning Disability and Other Related Issues

OMNIGRAPHICS
615 Griswold St., Ste. 520
Detroit, MI 48226

Library of Congress Cataloging-in-Publication Data

Names: Hayes, Kevin (Editor of health information), editor.

Title: Learning disabilities information for teens: health tips about academic skills disorders and other disabilities that affect learning including information about common signs of learning disabilities, school issues, learning to live with a learning disability, and other related issues / Kevin Hayes, editor.

Description: Third edition. | Detroit: Omnigraphics, Inc., [2020] | Series: Teen health series | Includes bibliographical references and index. | Audience: Ages 13 | Audience: Grades 7-9 | Summary: "Provides basic consumer health information for teens on identifying, diagnosing and living with various types of learning disabilities. Includes an index, and a directory of organizations to provide help or support for those with learning disabilities"-- Provided by publisher.

Identifiers: LCCN 2020023557 (print) | LCCN 2020023558 (ebook) | ISBN 9780780818149 (library binding) | ISBN 9780780818156 (ebook)

Subjects: LCSH: Learning disabilities--Health aspects.

Classification: LCC RJ496.L4 L434 2020 (print) | LCC RJ496.L4 (ebook) | DDC 618.92/85889--dc23

LC record available at https://lccn.loc.gov/2020023557

LC ebook record available at https://lccn.loc.gov/2020023558

TABLE OF CONTENTS

Part 3 | Congenital and Genetic Disorders That Affect Learning

Part 4 | Other Disabilities and Chronic Conditions That Impact Learning

Part 5 | School Options for Teens with Learning Disability

Part 6 | Career Options and Employment Support

Part 7 | Living with a Learning Disability

Part 8 | If You Need More Help or Information

PREFACE

About This Book

In the United States, nearly 7.1 million children and youth ages 3–21 in the year 2018–19 received special education services for learning disabilities, such as dyslexia, dyscalculia, and other disorders that affect language development, motor control, attention, and behavior. It is important to understand how students with learning disabilities can be helped. According to the 2019 *Building a Grad Nation Data Brief*, in 2017, the national graduation rate reached an all-time high of 84.6 percent, compared with just 67.1 percent of students with disabilities—a gap of more than 17.5 percentage points. Although most states saw improvements in their on-time graduation rate for students with disabilities, just 26 states saw increases of at least 1 percentage point. Moreover, 14 states saw their rates decline over the past year. Identifying and addressing problems as early as possible enables students to develop the skills and coping strategies needed to succeed in school and beyond.

Learning Disabilities Information for Teens, Third Edition describes the process of learning, the different kinds of learning disabilities, and their common signs, causes, and diagnostic procedures. It also discusses how other disabilities, disorders, and chronic conditions can affect learning. Information on academic issues, career options, and employment supports for young adults with learning disabilities is provided. Coping tips such as learning environments, assistive technology, and other adolescent issues along with facts about laws designed to protect the rights of people with learning disabilities are included. The book concludes with a directory of resources for further help and information.

How to Use This Book

This book is divided into parts and chapters. Parts focus on broad areas of interest; chapters are devoted to single topics within a part.

Part 1: Process of Learning: An Overview defines the learning process and provides information about gifted students with learning disabilities. It describes common signs and conditions associated with people with learning disabilities. Early intervention, statistics, and research on learning disabilities are discussed. Information on early learning, early literacy, and early education is also provided.

Part 2: Types of Learning Disabilities describes the categories of learning disabilities—ADHD, academic skills disorders, developmental speech and language disorders, and other disorders that include impaired sensory and motor skills, and information processing issues. The often-overlooked disruption in the executive function is also discussed.

Part 3: Congenital and Genetic Disorders That Affect Learning provides information on certain genetics and substance abuse disorders such as fetal alcohol spectrum disorders (FASDs), Down syndrome, Klinefelter syndrome, Turner syndrome, 47,XYY syndrome, Aarskog-Scott syndrome, Smith-Kingsmore syndrome, and Triple X syndrome.

Part 4: Other Disabilities and Chronic Conditions That Affect Learning provides information on medical conditions and physical challenges that can affect a student's ability to learn either by interrupting the educational process or by affecting the ways in which the brain processes information. These conditions include bipolar disorder, cancer treatment, aphasia, cerebral palsy, epilepsy, autism, Tourette syndrome, hearing loss, and pediatric sleep-disordered breathing.

Part 5: School Options for Teens with Learning Disability provides facts about understanding and accessing different school options. It explains how to choose a school, why special education services are important, and how to prepare for school-based experiences. It provides practical suggestions for areas such as educational options after high school, postsecondary education, and connecting activities to gain access to the chosen postschool option.

Part 6: Career Options and Employment Support provides information on transition planning, explains career development options, and offers tips about youth development and leadership and vocational rehabilitation. It also covers disability disclosure, volunteerism and service-learning, employment supports, a career with the federal government, and employers' efforts in finding, accommodating, and retaining employees with disabilities.

Part 7: Living with a Learning Disability offers help to students by providing information about deeper learning, service-learning, school supportive environment, and assistive technology. It also helps students in areas where they may face challenges, such as self-esteem, self-advocacy, and social skills. Commonly encountered problems, such as bullying, coping with sibling issues, barriers to participation, and employment discrimination, are also discussed. It also provides information on the laws that protect people with learning disabilities.

Part 8: If You Need More Information provides a directory of organizations that offer additional help and support.

Bibliographic Note

This volume contains documents and excerpts from publications issued by the following U.S. government agencies: Administration for Children and Families (ACF); Centers for Disease Control and Prevention (CDC); Corporation for National and Community Service (CNCS); *Eunice Kennedy Shriver* National Institute of Child Health and Human Development (NICHD); Genetic and Rare Diseases Information Center (GARD); Genetics Home Reference (GHR); Literacy Information and Communication System (LINCS); National Cancer Institute (NCI); National Institute of Mental Health (NIMH); National Institute of Neurological Disorders and Stroke (NINDS); National Institute on Deafness and Other Communication Disorders (NIDCD); National Institute on Disability, Independent Living, and Rehabilitation Research (NIDILRR); National Institutes of Health (NIH); U.S. Department of Education (ED); U.S. Department of Health and Human Services (HHS); U.S. Department of Labor (DOL); U.S. Department of Veterans Affairs (VA); U.S. Drug Enforcement Administration (DEA); U.S. Library of Congress (LOC); U.S. Social Security Administration (SSA); USA.gov; and Youth.gov.

It may also contain original material produced by Omnigraphics and reviewed by medical U.S. government agencies:

The photograph on the front cover is © fizkes/Shutterstock.

Medical Review

Omnigraphics contracts with a team of qualified, senior medical professionals who serve as medical consultants for the *Teen Health Series*. As necessary, medical consultants review reprinted and originally written material for currency and accuracy. Citations including the phrase "Reviewed (month, year)" indicate material reviewed by this team. Medical consultation services are provided to the *Teen Health Series* editors by:

Dr. Vijayalakshmi, MBBS, DGO, MD
Dr. Senthil Selvan, MBBS, DCH, MD
Dr. K. Sivanandham, MBBS, DCH, MS (Research), PhD

About The *Teen Health Series*

At the request of librarians serving today's teens and young adults, the *Teen Health Series* was developed as a specially focused set of volumes within Omnigraphics' *Health Reference Series*. Each volume deals comprehensively with a topic selected according to the needs and interests of people in middle school and high school. Teens seeking preventive guidance, information about disease warning signs, medical statistics, and risk factors for health problems will find answers to their questions in the *Teen Health Series*. The *Series*, however, is not intended to serve as a tool for diagnosing illness, in prescribing treatments, or as a substitute for the physician–patient relationship. All people concerned about medical symptoms or the possibility of disease are encouraged to seek professional care from an appropriate healthcare provider.

If there is a topic you would like to see addressed in a future volume of the *Teen Health Series*, please write to:

Managing Editor
Teen Health Series
Omnigraphics
615 Griswold St., Ste. 520
Detroit, MI 48226

A Note About Spelling And Style

Teen Health Series editors use *Stedman's Medical Dictionary* as an authority for questions related to the spelling of medical terms and *the Chicago Manual of Style* for questions related to grammatical structures, punctuation, and other editorial concerns. Consistent adherence is not always possible, however, because the individual volumes within the *Series* include many documents from a wide variety of different producers and copyright holders, and the editor's primary goal is to present material from each source as accurately as is possible following the terms specified by each document's producer. This sometimes means that information in different chapters may follow other guidelines and alternate spelling authorities. For example, occasionally a copyright holder may require that eponymous terms be shown in possessive forms (Crohn's disease vs. Crohn disease) or that British spelling norms be retained (leukaemia vs. leukemia).

PART 1 | PROCESS OF LEARNING: AN OVERVIEW

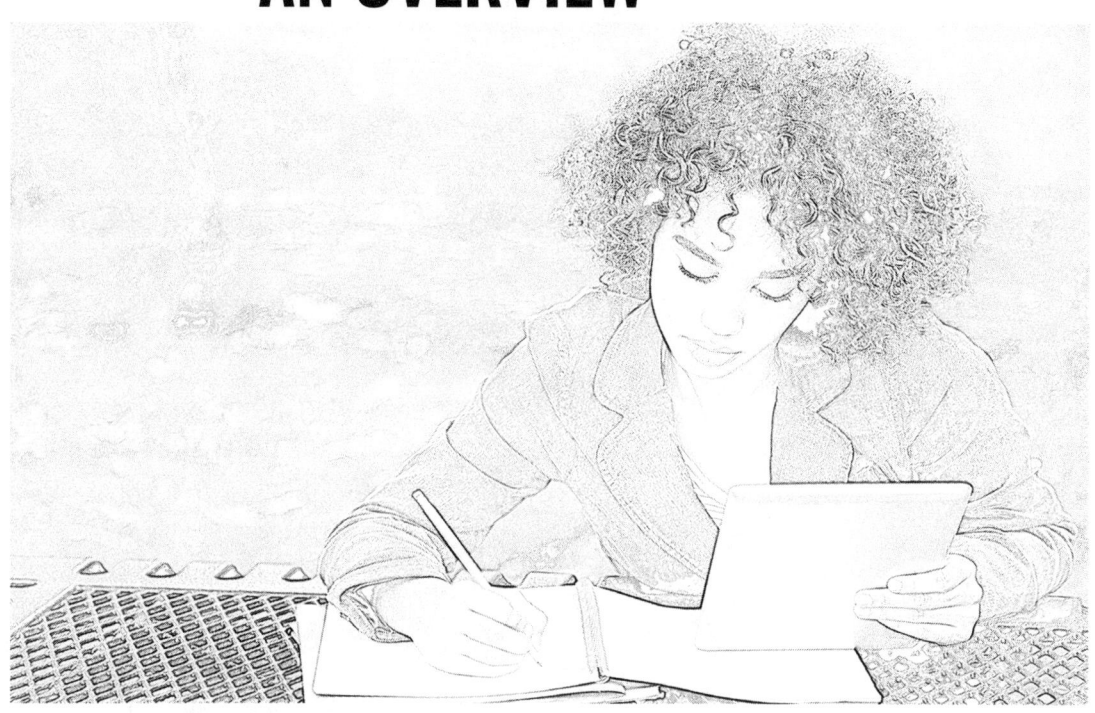

CHAPTER 1
LEARNING PROCESS

About This Chapter: This chapter includes text excerpted from "Early Learning," *Eunice Kennedy Shriver* National Institute of Child Health and Human Development (NICHD), December 1, 2016. Reviewed July 2020.

Learning begins in the womb. And, from the moment they are born, children begin interacting with the world around them and building critical skills. What they learn in their first few years of life—and how they learn it—can have long-lasting effects on their health and on their later success in school and in work.

"Early learning" refers to the skills and concepts that children develop before they reach kindergarten. It is a crucial part of development and can set patterns for both school and adult learning.

By studying early learning, researchers can figure out the best ways for parents and caregivers to encourage children to develop these skills and concepts and to put children on a path to becoming lifetime learners.

The *Eunice Kennedy Shriver* National Institute of Child Health and Human Development (NICHD) early learning research studies:

- Early social relationships with family, caretakers, teachers, and peers
- How children's environment, including exposure to stress and media, promotes or inhibits learning
- Ways to improve learning
- School readiness—effective ways to get children ready to participate and learn in a school classroom environment
- Long-term impact of early intervention programs
- How professional development of caretakers impacts learning

Why Is Early Learning Important?

Early learning paves the way for learning at school and throughout life. What children learn in their first few years of life—and how they learn it—can have long-lasting effects on their success and health as children, teens, and adults.

3

Studies show that supporting children's early learning can lead to:
- Higher test scores from preschool to age 21
- Better grades in reading and math
- A better chance of staying in school and going to college
- Fewer teen pregnancies
- Improved mental health
- Lower risk of heart disease in adulthood
- A longer lifespan

What Are Some Factors That Affect Early Learning?

A child's home, family, and daily life have a strong effect on her or his ability to learn. Parents and guardians can control some things in their child's life and environment, but not everything.

Some factors that can affect early learning include:
- Parents' education
- Family income
- The number of parents in the home
- Access to books and play materials
- Stability of home life
- Going to preschool
- Quality of childcare
- Stress levels and exposure to stress (in the womb, as an infant, and as a child)
- How many languages are spoken at home

Why Is It Important to Study Early Learning?

Early learning can improve children's health and well-being and have long-lasting benefits. Studying which factors affect early learning and education will help researchers:
- Design better ways to help at-risk children before they start school
- Improve parent, caregiver, childcare provider, and preschool teacher training
- Use research findings to design better preschool and childcare programs
- Study innovative early intervention settings, such as pediatrician's offices and home visitor programs, and ways to make these programs convenient for parents and caretakers.

For example, the NICHD research has helped characterize a positive learning environment as one with a warm caregiver and in which the child is supported and challenged cognitively. Findings of NICHD research also link early childhood education programs to improved adult health and demonstrate that early learning programs are cost-effective.

Recent examples include findings indicating that:

- Research shows that Head Start has positive effects on children's math, literacy, and vocabulary skills across the board. The program had an even greater impact—boosting early math skills most—among children whose parents spent little time reading to them or counting with them at home. Children whose homes provided a medium amount of such activities had the biggest gains in early literacy skills.
- Children who have trouble developing language skills may also have trouble controlling their impulses and behaviors.
- Bilingual speakers develop brain networks that help them filter out unnecessary information better than those who speak only one language. These brain networks might protect against Alzheimer disease and other age-related brain problems.
- Experience and genetic factors seem to influence whether a child will have "math anxiety"—very strong worries about math abilities that can be disabling.

How Can Parents and Caregivers Promote Early Learning?

A child's home, family, and daily life have a strong effect on her or his ability to learn.

You are your child's first teacher, and every day is filled with opportunities to help her or him learn. You can help by:

- Reading to your child, beginning when she or he is born
- Pointing out and talking with your child about the names, colors, shapes, numbers, sizes, and quantities of objects in her or his environment
- Listening and responding to your child as she or he learns to communicate
- Practicing counting together

CHAPTER 2
GIFTED STUDENTS WITH LEARNING DISABILITIES

How can a gifted student have a learning disability? At first glance, those seem like contradictory terms. And, indeed, when educators first began identifying a subgroup of students who exhibited both outstanding intellectual ability and learning disabilities, even some experts were skeptical. Yet research has found that about 14 percent of children classified as gifted might also have learning problems, compared to around four percent of all children.

But, unfortunately, not all teachers are trained to identify these co-occurring phenomena, and in some states, programs are available to help either gifted children or those with learning disabilities, but not both. As a result, many students have been unable to get the specialized help they need. Luckily, the picture is changing as this issue is becoming better understood. More research is being done, new publications are appearing all the time, and many educational conferences now include sessions devoted to the topic.

Who Are Students with Learning Disabilities?

Gifted students with learning disabilities—often called "Gifted/LD," "double-labeled," or "twice exceptional" by educators—are those who exhibit extraordinary talent in some areas of academic achievement and disabling weaknesses in others. Because of their puzzling, inconsistent performance in school, they tend to be among the most

Gifted students may have underlying learning disabilities that include Asperger syndrome (AS), attention deficit disorder (ADD), attention deficit hyperactivity disorder (ADHD), and physical or emotional problems. In some cases when these disorders are identified, the student's gifted abilities may be overlooked.

misunderstood and misdiagnosed individuals in the student population, so they frequently fall through the cracks in the system and never get the type of attention they need. Many experts classify these students into three main groups:

- **Students who have been identified as gifted yet have difficulty at school.** These students have been identified as gifted by virtue of their IQ score, performance on standardized tests, or achievement in certain academic areas. But, since they underperform in other areas, they are often mislabeled as "underachievers" or are simply called "lazy."
- **Those with an identified learning disability, but whose intellectual ability has gone unnoticed.** Because this group of students struggle profoundly in school, their disability is readily apparent to educators and parents. But, because efforts to help them focus only on correcting the disability, their talents may never be uncovered. As a result, their self-esteem suffers, they may become discouraged, and they might never reach their full potential in those areas in which they could succeed.
- **Students not classified as either gifted or learning disabled.** In a sense, these students' strengths and weaknesses cancel each other out, and they perform at an average grade level. Because they are doing well enough, their problems and abilities are not recognized, and they do not qualify for the special help they require in either area. Although grade-level performance may be adequate, this group of students has the potential for much higher achievement, but without the proper attention they might never get the chance to excel.

Identifying Students Who Are Both Gifted and Learning Disabled

Because the characteristics of Gifted/LD students vary from individual to individual, and because they are so often misunderstood, it can be difficult to identify them and address their needs. But, there are a number of indicators they often have in common. A few of these include:

- Unexplained inconsistent academic performance
- High achievement in complex interests outside of school
- Excellent verbal skills but difficulty with written language
- Difficulty with memorization, but good at complex analysis
- Excelling at one type of test (e.g., multiple choice) but doing poorly on another
- Wander off-task frequently and daydream or become disruptive
- Concentrate for long periods on tasks they find interesting but become bored when a subject does not interest them

Helping Gifted Students with Learning Disabilities

The first steps in helping Gifted/LD students are to increase teacher education and community awareness and to expand special-needs programs to include curricula for these students. At the moment, many government and community programs do not include Gifted/LD children, and many school systems are not equipped to address their needs. Other suggestions include:

- Focus on the child's gift, not just the disability.
- Encourage students to choose tasks that rely on their strengths.
- Recognize and encourage individual learning styles.
- Stress concepts first, then details.
- Establish concrete goals, and celebrate successes.
- Provide accelerated coursework in gifted areas, remedial work for weak areas.
- Connect new lessons to past learning, and provide rationale for tasks.
- Help students develop compensation strategies for disabilities.
- Recognize student frustration, and allow them to withdraw from activities with dignity.
- Teach through discussion and inquiry, rather than rote memorization.
- Connect lessons to the world beyond the classroom.
- Establish individual, peer, and group counseling sessions.
- Promote self-awareness to help students develop their own learning strategies.
- Create a nurturing environment that values individual differences.
- Encourage interests outside of school that make use of special talents.
- Establish awareness, education, and support programs for parents, coaches, and other adults who are in regular contact with these students.
- Gifted students with learning disabilities have the potential to achieve classroom success, become enthusiastic learners, develop self-confidence, and gain the knowledge they need to be their own advocates throughout their lifetimes. But, this will only happen through increased awareness on the part of teachers, parents, and the community, and through specialized educational programs designed to meet their needs.

References

1. Brody, Linda E.; Carol J. Mills. "Gifted Children with Learning Disabilities: A Review of the Issues," LD Online, 1997.
2. Douglass, Marcy J. "Twice Exceptional: Gifted Students with Learning Disabilities," WM.edu, May 2007.
3. Perras, Cindy, M.Ed. "Gifted Students with LDs: What Teachers Need to Know," LDatSchool.ca, February 18, 2015.
4. Shenfield, Tali, CPsych. "Helping Gifted Students with Learning Disability," Psy-Ed.com, October 18, 2016.
5. Wormald, Catherine. "Intellectually Gifted Students Often Have Learning Disabilities," TheConversation.com, March 24, 2015.

CHAPTER 3
EARLY LITERACY

About This Chapter: This chapter includes text excerpted from "Early Beginnings," Literacy Information and Communication System (LINCS), U.S. Department of Education (ED), January 15, 2009. Reviewed July 2020.

Learning and Development in the Preschool Years

The years from birth through age 5 are a critical time for children's development and learning. Early childhood educators understand that at home and in early childhood education settings, young children learn important skills that can provide them with the cornerstones needed for the development of later academic skills. Research confirms that patterns of learning in preschool are closely linked to later achievement: children who develop more skills in the preschool years perform better in the primary grades. The development of early skills appears to be particularly important in the area of literacy. It is estimated that more than a third of all American fourth-graders (and an even higher percentage of our at-risk students) read so poorly that they cannot complete their schoolwork successfully. Providing young children with the critical precursor skills to reading can offer a path to improving overall achievement.

Connection between Early Literacy Skills and How Children Learn to Be Readers, Writers, and Spellers

Early literacy skills have a clear and consistently strong relationship with later conventional literacy skills, such as decoding, oral reading, fluency, reading comprehension, writing, and spelling. Even before children start school, they can become aware of systematic patterns of sounds in spoken language, manipulate sounds in words, recognize words and break them apart into smaller units, learn the relationship between sounds and letters, and build their oral language and vocabulary skills. These are all skills that the National Early Literacy Panel found to be precursors to children's later growth in the ability to decode and comprehend text, to write, and to spell. Although there is evidence of a link between early literacy and later developing literacy skills, some early literacy skills appear to be more important than others. The strongest and

11

most consistent predictors of later literacy development are alphabet knowledge, phonological awareness and memory, rapid automatized naming of letters and objects, and writing letters. There are other early foundational skills that also can make a difference in getting children ready for the next step...for learning how to read.

Early Literacy Guide

Early literacy skills are sometimes called "emergent," "precursor," "foundational," or "predictive" literacy skills to distinguish them from more conventional literacy skills, such as decoding, oral reading, fluency, reading comprehension, writing, and spelling.

Literacy

All the activities involved in speaking, listening, reading, writing, and appreciating both spoken and written language.

Early Literacy Skills

Skills that begin to develop in the preschool years, such as alphabet knowledge, phonological awareness, letter writing, print knowledge, and oral language.

- **Alphabet knowledge.** Knowing the names and sounds associated with printed letters.
- **Concepts (conventions) about print.** The knowledge of print conventions (e.g., left-right, front-back) and concepts (e.g., book cover, author, and text).
- **Conventional literacy skills.** More mature skills such as decoding, oral reading, fluency, reading comprehension, writing, and spelling that are the focus of instruction in elementary and secondary school students.
- **Decoding.** The ability to apply knowledge of letter-sound relationships, including knowledge of letter patterns, to correctly pronounce written words.
- **Environmental print.** The print of everyday life, such as the letters, numbers, shapes, and colors found in logos and signs for products and stores (e.g., Coke and McDonald's).
- **Onset-rime.** Parts of monosyllabic words in spoken language that are smaller than syllables—onset is the initial consonant sound of a syllable (the onset of 'bag' is 'b'); rime is the part of a syllable that contains the vowel and all that follows it (the rime of 'bag' is '-ag').
- **Oral language.** The ability to produce or comprehend spoken language, including vocabulary or grammar.
- **Oral reading fluency.** The ability to accurately and quickly read a series of words or sentences.
- **Phoneme.** The smallest unit of sound that changes the meanings of spoken words (e.g., by changing the first phoneme in bat from /b/ to /p/, the word 'bat' changes to 'pat').

- **Phonological awareness.** The ability to detect, manipulate, or analyze the auditory aspects of spoken language (including the ability to distinguish or segment words, syllables, or phonemes) independent of meaning.
- **Phonological memory.** The ability to remember spoken information for a short period of time.
- **Print knowledge.** A skill reflecting a combination of elements of alphabet knowledge, concepts about print, and early decoding.
- **Rapid automatized naming.** The ability to name rapidly a sequence of random letters, digits, objects, or colors.
- **Reading comprehension.** The ability to understand and gain meaning from text.
- **Syllable.** A part of a word that contains a vowel or, in spoken language, a vowel sound (e.g., e-vent, news-pa-per).
- **Visual processing.** The ability to match or discriminate visually presented symbols.

CHAPTER 4
EARLY CHILDHOOD EDUCATION

About This Chapter: This chapter includes text excerpted from "Early Childhood Education," Centers for Disease Control and Prevention (CDC), August 5, 2016. Reviewed July 2020.

What Is Early Childhood Education?

Early childhood education (ECE) aims to improve the cognitive and social development of children ages 3 or 4 years. ECE interventions can improve all children's development and act as a protective factor against the future onset of adult disease and disability. Children disadvantaged by poverty may experience an even greater benefit because ECE programs also seek to prevent or minimize gaps in school readiness between low-income and more economically advantaged children.

All ECE programs must address one or more of the following: literacy, numeracy, cognitive development, socioemotional development, and motor skills. Some programs may offer additional components, including recreation, meals, healthcare, parental supports, and social services. ECE programs may be delivered in a variety of ways and settings. State and district programs may be available to all children regardless of income. For example, Georgia and Oklahoma have implemented universal preschool programs for all 4-year-olds. Other programs, including federally funded Head Start and evidence-based model programs, such as the Abecedarian and Perry Preschool programs, are provided specifically for low-income and at-risk children. The Child-Parent Center (CPC) program is another example of a widely-implemented model program; it expanded into 33 sites in Minnesota, Wisconsin, and Illinois through a University of Minnesota project funded by the U.S. Department of Education (ED).

What Is the Public-Health Issue?

Childhood development is an important determinant of health over a person's lifetime. Early developmental opportunities can provide a foundation for children's academic success, health, and general well-being. Preschool-aged children experience profound biological brain development and achieve 90 percent of their adult brain volume by age 6. This physiological growth allows children to develop functional skills related to information processing, comprehension, language, emotional regulation, and motor skills. Experiences during early childhood affect the structural development of the brain and the neurobiological pathways that determine a child's functional development.

Positive experiences support children's cognitive, social, emotional, and physical development, and conversely, adverse experiences can hinder it. Additionally, strong associations have been found between the biological effects of adverse early childhood experiences and numerous adult diseases, including coronary artery disease, chronic pulmonary disease, and cancer.

Children in low-income families often are exposed to more adverse early childhood experiences and environmental factors that delay or compromise their development and place them at a disadvantage for healthy growth and school readiness. In the United States, 15.5 million children (21%) lived in families with incomes below 100 percent Federal Poverty Level (FPL) in 2010. Also in 2010, less than half of children in families in the lowest income quartile were enrolled in center-based early childhood education programs.

What Is the Evidence of Health Impact and Cost-Effectiveness?

Early childhood education interventions can improve children's development and act as a protective factor against the future onset of adult disease and disability. ECE can counteract the disadvantage some children experience, improve their social and cognitive development, and provide them with an equal opportunity to achieve school readiness, and lifelong employment, income, and health. Systematic reviews of studies examining the effects of three types of center-based ECE programs, found that they were associated with:

- Improved cognitive development
- Improved emotional development
- Improved self-regulation
- Improved academic achievement

ECE benefit estimates, both short- and long-term, included some or all of the following major components:

- Increases in maternal employment and income
- Reductions in crime, welfare dependency, and child abuse and neglect
- Savings from reduced grade retention
- Savings in healthcare costs
- Savings in remedial education and child care costs
- Improvement in health outcomes associated with education
- Earnings gains associated with high school graduation
- Better jobs and higher earnings throughout employment years for children participating in these programs

Additional studies have found that ECE is associated with other positive health effects, including healthier weight (such as fewer underweight, overweight, and obese children).

A recent systematic economic review found that the economic benefits exceed costs for different types of ECE programs. Based on earnings gains alone, the benefit-to-cost ratios ranged from:

- 3.06:1 to 5.19:1 for State and District programs
- 1.58:1 to 2.51:1 for Federal Head Start programs
- 1.76:1 to 4.39:1 for model programs

The rate of return on investment was much higher when all benefit components including earnings gains were considered. For model programs, based on total benefits, the return on every dollar invested was:

- $2.49 for the Abecedarian program
- $8.60 for the Perry Preschool
- $10.83 for Chicago Child-Parent Center

CHAPTER 5
EARLY LEARNING AND SCHOOL READINESS PROGRAM

About This Chapter: This chapter includes text excerpted from "CDBB Research Programs," *Eunice Kennedy Shriver* National Institute of Child Health and Human Development (NICHD), June 10, 2019.

Early learning and school readiness program supports basic and translational developmental research that attempts to specify the experiences children need from birth to 8 years of age to prepare them for a successful transition to school entry and later achievement. It also supports long-term follow-up studies that quantify the long-term effect of early intervention programs. School readiness encompasses those capabilities of children, families, schools, and communities that will best foster student success in kindergarten and beyond. The components of school readiness include physical growth and well-being; motor, cognitive, socioemotional, and executive function/self-regulation skill development; and emergent language, literacy, numeracy, and mathematics learning.

Developmentally Informed Prevention and Early Intervention Studies

Studies of basic and translational genetic, epigenetic, and neurodevelopmental processes and mechanisms that underlie cognitive, executive function, language, social, emotional, motor, or physical development in the context of applying this knowledge to guide the development and testing of prevention and early intervention studies whose primary outcome is the promotion of early learning and the development of school readiness skills and abilities in at-risk populations.

Early Social Interactions

Basic and translational research is supported to identify the mechanisms through which early interactions with family members, adult caretakers, teachers, and peers in a variety of early care and education settings support learning and school readiness in children from diverse backgrounds and environments.

Environmental Impacts

Research that specifies the mechanisms by which environmental variables, such as exposure to high levels of stress, chaotic or otherwise, over- and under-stimulating environments, and inappropriate exposure to media negatively affect children's early learning and the development of school readiness skills and abilities.

Infant/Toddler Interventions

Interest in the development and testing of targeted and comprehensive intervention programs for at-risk infants and toddlers ages 0 to 2 and their families that are delivered in the home and/or in-service settings such as pediatric primary care clinics, family- and center-based childcare settings, and Early Head Start programs whose primary focus is the promotion of early learning and the development of school readiness skills and abilities.

Preschooler Interventions

Interest in the development and testing of integrative and comprehensive early childhood education interventions for at-risk children, ages three to five, that are delivered in early care and education programs such as Head Start and state and local preschool programs and center-based childcare providers whose primary focus is the promotion of early learning and the development of school readiness skills and abilities. Interventions may be designed to target specific subpopulations of children and their families, including children who are English-language learners.

Professional Development Linked to Child Outcomes

Knowledge about the preparation, training, and professional development of people involved in the care and education of young children, the effectiveness of training strategies in promoting the positive modes of interaction identified by the research previously described, and the causal linkages between adult behavior and school readiness outcomes for young children.

Measurement Development

New and innovative methods and assessments for measuring early learning and school readiness skills and abilities in diverse populations of children as well as measures of home, childcare, and preschool environments and practices that are related to child learning and development.

CHAPTER 6
WHAT IS A LEARNING DISABILITY?

About This Chapter: This chapter includes text excerpted from "About Learning Disabilities," *Eunice Kennedy Shriver* National Institute of Child Health and Human Development (NICHD), September 11, 2018.

Learning disabilities affect how a person learns to read, write, speak, and do math. They are caused by differences in the brain, most often in how it functions but also sometimes in its structure. These differences affect the way the brain processes information.

Learning disabilities are often discovered once a child is in school and has learning difficulties that do not improve over time. A person can have more than one learning disability. Learning disabilities can last a person's entire life, but she or he can still be successful with the right educational supports.

Types of Learning Disabilities
Some of the most common learning disabilities are the following:
- **Dyslexia.** People with dyslexia have problems with reading words accurately and with ease (sometimes called "fluency") and may have a hard time spelling, understanding sentences, and recognizing words they already know.
- **Dysgraphia.** People with dysgraphia have problems with their handwriting. They may have trouble forming letters, writing within a defined space, and writing down their thoughts.
- **Dyscalculia.** People with this math learning disability may have difficulty understanding arithmetic concepts and doing addition, multiplication, and measuring.

A learning disability is not an indication of a person's intelligence. Learning disabilities are different from learning problems due to intellectual and developmental disabilities, or emotional, vision, hearing, or motor skills problems.

- **Apraxia of speech.** This disorder involves problems with speaking. People with this disorder have trouble saying what they want to say. It is sometimes called "verbal apraxia."
- **Central auditory processing disorder.** People with this condition have trouble understanding and remembering language-related tasks. They have difficulty explaining things, understanding jokes, and following directions. They confuse words and are easily distracted.
- **Nonverbal learning disorders.** People with these conditions have strong verbal skills but difficulty understanding facial expression and body language. They are clumsy and have trouble generalizing and following multistep directions.

Because there are many different types of learning disabilities, and some people may have more than one, it is hard to estimate how many people might have learning disabilities.

CHAPTER 7
WHAT ARE SOME COMMON SIGNS OF LEARNING DISABILITIES?

About This Chapter: Text in this chapter begins with excerpts from "What Are Some Signs of Learning Disabilities?" *Eunice Kennedy Shriver* National Institute of Child Health and Human Development (NICHD), September 11, 2018; Text under the heading "What Causes Learning Disabilities" is excerpted from "What Causes Learning Disabilities?" *Eunice Kennedy Shriver* National Institute of Child Health and Human Development (NICHD), September 11, 2018; Text under the heading "How Are Learning Disabilities Diagnosed?" © 2016 Omnigraphics. Reviewed July 2020.

Many children have trouble reading, writing, or performing other learning-related tasks at some point. This does not mean they have learning disabilities (LDs). A child with an LD often has several related signs, and they do not go away or get better over time. The signs of LDs vary from person to person.

Please note that the generally common signs included here are for informational purposes only; the information is not intended to screen for LDs in general or for a specific type of LD.

Common Signs of Learning Disabilities
Common signs that a person may have LDs include the following:
- Problems reading and/or writing
- Problems with math
- Poor memory
- Problems paying attention
- Trouble following directions
- Clumsiness
- Trouble telling time
- Problems staying organized

A child with an LD also may have one or more of the following:
- Acting without really thinking about possible outcomes (impulsiveness)
- "Acting out" in school or social situations
- Difficulty staying focused; being easily distracted
- Difficulty saying a word correctly out loud or expressing thoughts
- Problems with school performance from week to week or day to day
- Speaking such as a younger child; using short, simple phrases; or leaving out words in sentences
- Having a hard time listening
- Problems dealing with changes in schedule or situations
- Problems understanding words or concepts

These signs alone are not enough to determine that a person has an LD. Only a professional can diagnose an LD.

Each LD has its own signs. A person with a particular disability may not have all of the signs of that disability.

Children being taught in a second language may show signs of learning problems or an LD. The LD assessment must take into account whether a student is bilingual or a second language learner. In addition, for English-speaking children, the assessment should be sensitive to differences that may be due to dialect, a form of a language that is specific to a region or group.

Below are some common LDs and the signs associated with them:

Dyslexia

People with dyslexia usually have trouble making the connection between letters and sounds and with spelling and recognizing words.

People with dyslexia often show other signs of the condition. These may include:
- Having a hard time understanding what others are saying
- Difficulty organizing written and spoken language
- Delay in being able to speak
- Difficulty expressing thoughts or feelings
- Difficulty learning new words (vocabulary), either while reading or hearing
- Trouble learning foreign languages
- Difficulty learning songs and rhymes
- Slow rate of reading, both silently and out loud
- Giving up on longer reading tasks
- Difficulty understanding questions and following directions
- Poor spelling
- Problems remembering numbers in sequence (e.g., telephone numbers and addresses)
- Trouble telling left from right

Dysgraphia

A child who has trouble writing or has very poor handwriting and does not outgrow it may have dysgraphia. This disorder may cause a child to be tense and twist awkwardly when holding a pen or pencil.

Other signs of this condition may include:

- A strong dislike of writing and/or drawing
- Problems with grammar
- Trouble writing down ideas
- Losing energy or interest as soon as they start writing
- Trouble writing down thoughts in a logical sequence
- Saying words out loud while writing
- Leaving words unfinished or omitting them when writing sentences

Dyscalculia

Signs of this disability include problems understanding basic arithmetic concepts, such as fractions, number lines, and positive and negative numbers.

Other symptoms may include:

- Difficulty with math-related word problems
- Trouble making change in cash transactions
- Messiness in putting math problems on paper
- Trouble with logical sequences (e.g., steps in math problems)
- Trouble understanding the time sequence of events
- Trouble describing math processes

What Causes Learning Disabilities

Researchers do not know all of the possible causes of LDs, but they have found a range of risk factors during their work to find potential causes. Research shows that risk factors may be present from birth and tend to run in families. In fact, children who have a parent with an LD are more likely to develop an LD themselves. To better understand LDs, researchers are studying how children's brains learn to read, write, and develop math skills. Researchers are working on interventions to help address the needs of those who struggle with reading the most, including those with LDs, to improve learning and overall health.

Factors that affect a fetus developing in the womb, such as alcohol or drug use, can put a child at higher risk for a learning problem or disability. Other factors in an infant's environment may play a role, too. These can include poor nutrition or exposure to lead in water or in paint. Young children who do not receive the support they need for their intellectual development may show signs of LDs once they start school.

Sometimes a person may develop an LD later in life due to injury. Possible causes in such a case include dementia or a traumatic brain injury (TBI).

Alcohol can cause alterations in the structure and function of the developing brain, which continues to mature into a person's mid-20s, and it may have consequences reaching far beyond adolescence.

In adolescence, brain development is characterized by dramatic changes to the brain's structure, neuron connectivity (i.e., "wiring"), and physiology. These changes in the brain affect everything from emerging sexuality to emotionality and judgment.

(Source: "Alcohol and the Developing Brain," Substance Abuse and Mental Health Services Administration (SAMHSA))

How Are Learning Disabilities Diagnosed?

Diagnosing LDs is difficult because LDs show up differently in different people and an LD in one area may be masked by accelerated ability in another. For instance, a child who has dyscalculia may not know how to add two numbers, but may write at a much higher grade level, leading teachers to think she or he is just being lazy about turning in her or his math homework.

Diagnosing Learning Disabilities in School-Aged Children and Adolescents

Learning disabilities often become evident when a child starts school. Teachers and other school professionals may identify students with suspected LDs as they monitor the students' progress and their response to educational assistance. This is called the "response to intervention" (RTI) process. Parents may also bring their concerns about LDs in their children to the attention of school professionals.

If a student is suspected of having LDs, further testing and evaluation will be needed.

The Individuals with Disabilities Education Act (IDEA) sets out clear rules and regulations on the process for evaluating children suspected of having LDs, so that students with LDs can take advantage of individualized educational plans (IEPs) when warranted. Under IDEA, an evaluation must be "full and individual" meaning it needs to be comprehensive in scope but tailored to the student as a distinct individual. Tests must be given in the language and at the level that the student understands best. Tests must investigate all the skills where the student has difficulty. The results must give relevant information to make informed decisions on the next steps in the student's educational plan.

In addition, the school staff must create an evaluation plan that informs the parents of all tests, observations, records they plan to use in the evaluation as well as providing the names of all evaluators.

The evaluation may include:

- **A physical examination** that looks for physical causes of LD such as vision, hearing, movement, or other health issues.
- **A psychological evaluation** to examine the student's emotional health and social skills, and determine how the student learns best.

What Does It Mean

The Individuals with Disabilities Education Act (IDEA) is a law ensuring services to children with disabilities throughout the nation. IDEA governs how states and public agencies provide early intervention, special education and related services to more than 6.5 million eligible infants, toddlers, children, and youth with disabilities.

The Individualized Education Program (IEP) creates an opportunity for teachers, parents, school administrators, related services personnel, and students (when appropriate) to work together to improve educational results for children with disabilities. The IEP is the cornerstone of a quality education for each child with a disability.

(Sources: "Building the Legacy: IDEA 2004," U.S. Department of Education (ED); "A Guide to the Individualized Education Program," U.S. Department of Education (ED))

- **Interviews** with the student, parents, and teachers to learn more about the student's academic history, behavior in and out of school, and other information that can help the evaluators with their diagnosis.
- **Behavioral assessment** is often accomplished using questionnaires filled out by teachers and parents about how the student interacts with the world in both normal and unusual situations.
- **Observation of the student** by teachers, the school psychologist, reading specialist, speech-language pathologist, and other educational professionals.
- **Standardized tests that** are selected by educational professionals based on the student's areas of strengths and weaknesses. These tests can test general ability or specific skills.
  - *Intelligence and achievement tests* are used to measure the student's intellectual potential, what she or he knows and can do, and areas of the student's strengths and weaknesses. There are a variety of standard intelligence and achievement tests geared to a person's age. The evaluators then use the results of these tests to focus on what further testing needs to done.
  - *Tests for reading, writing, and math* can include those that measure reading comprehension to determine the grade level at which a student should be taught; essential reading skills; oral reading (can the student read a passage aloud then answer questions on it?); pronunciation; general math skills.
  - *Tests for language, motor, and processing skills* look at issues that affect a student's learning skills. Results of this type of test may suggest problems with perception, memory, planning, motor skills, attention, and comprehension of both written and spoken communications.
- **Other information already on file** including report cards and state test scores.

Based on the results of the evaluation, the school's IEP administrator will work with the student's teachers and family to draw up a plan of study to accommodate the student's LDs and determine strategies for effective learning and living.

References

1. "Adult Learning Disability Assessment Process," Learning Disabilities Association of America (LDA), 2016.
2. "Adults with Learning Disabilities—An Overview," Learning Disabilities Association of America (LDA), 2016.
3. "How Are Learning Disabilities Diagnosed?" *Eunice Kennedy Shriver* National Institute of Child Health and Human Development (NICHD), February 28, 2014.
4. Griffin, Rayma. "Who Can Diagnose Learning and Attention Issues in Adults?" Understood.org, 2016.
5. Morin, Amanda. "Understanding the Full Evaluation Process," Understood. org, July 11, 2014.
6. Patino, Erica. "Types of Behavior Assessments," Understood.org, May 30, 2014.
7. Patino, Erica. "Types of Intelligence and Achievement Tests," Understood.org, June 5, 2014.
8. Patino, Erica. "Types of Tests for Language, Motor and Processing Skills," Understood.org, June 5, 2014.
9. Patino, Erica. "Types of Tests for Reading, Writing and Math," Understood.org, November 18, 2014.

CHAPTER 8

DETERMINING THE EXISTENCE OF A SPECIFIC LEARNING DISABILITY FOR K-12

About This Chapter: This chapter includes text excerpted from "Sec. 300.309 Determining the Existence of a Specific Learning Disability," U.S. Department of Education (ED), May 25, 2018.

Specific Learning Disability Determination

The group described in §300.306 of Individuals with Disabilities Education Act (IDEA) may determine that a child has a specific learning disability, as defined in §300.8(c)(10) of IDEA as follows.

Does Not Achieve Adequately

The child does not achieve adequately for the child's age or to meet State-approved grade-level standards in one or more of the following areas, when provided with learning experiences and instruction appropriate for the child's age or State-approved grade-level standards:

- Oral expression
- Listening comprehension
- Written expression
- Basic reading skill
- Reading fluency skills
- Reading comprehension
- Mathematics calculation
- Mathematics problem solving

Does Not Make Sufficient Progress

The child does not make sufficient progress to meet age or State-approved grade-level standards in one or more of the areas identified in the above heading when using a process based on the child's response to scientific, research-based intervention.

Or, the child exhibits a pattern of strengths and weaknesses in performance, achievement, or both, relative to age, State-approved grade-level standards, or intellectual development, that is determined by the group to be relevant to the identification of a specific learning disability, using appropriate assessments, consistent with §§300.304 and 300.305 of IDEA.

Other Findings

The group determines that its findings under the two above headings are not primarily the result of:

- A visual, hearing, or motor disability
- An intellectual disability
- Emotional disturbance
- Cultural factors
- Environmental or economic disadvantage
- Limited English proficiency

Specific Learning Disability Is Not Due to Lack of Appropriate Instruction in Reading or Math

To ensure that underachievement in a child suspected of having a specific learning disability is not due to lack of appropriate instruction in reading or math, the group must consider, as part of the evaluation described in §§300.304 through 300.306 of IDEA.

1. Data that demonstrate that prior to, or as a part of, the referral process, the child was provided appropriate instruction in regular education settings, delivered by qualified personnel.
2. Data-based documentation of repeated assessments of achievement at reasonable intervals, reflecting formal assessment of student progress during instruction, which was provided to the child's parents.

Parental Consent

The public agency must promptly request parental consent to evaluate the child to determine if the child needs special education and related services, and must adhere to the timeframes described in §§300.301 and 300.303 of IDEA, unless extended by mutual written agreement of the child's parents and a group of qualified professionals, as described in §300.306(a)(1) of IDEA.

1. If, prior to a referral, a child has not made adequate progress after an appropriate period of time when provided instruction, as described in the above heading.
2. Whenever a child is referred for an evaluation.

CHAPTER 9
EARLY INTERVENTION FOR LEARNING DISABILITIES

About This Chapter: This chapter includes text excerpted from "Learning Disabilities—What Are the Treatments for Learning Disabilities?" *Eunice Kennedy Shriver* National Institute of Child Health and Human Development (NICHD), September 11, 2018.

Learning disabilities have no cure, but early intervention can lessen their effects. People with learning disabilities can develop ways to cope with their disabilities. Getting help earlier increases the chance of success in school and later in life. If learning disabilities remain untreated, a child may begin to feel frustrated, which can lead to low self-esteem and other problems.

Experts can help a child learn skills by building on the child's strengths and finding ways to compensate for the child's weaknesses. Interventions vary depending on the nature and extent of the disability.

Special Education Services

Children diagnosed with learning disabilities can receive special education services. The Individuals with Disabilities Education Act (IDEA) requires that public schools provide free special education support to children with disabilities.

In most states, each child is entitled to these services beginning at age three years and extending through high school or until age 21, whichever comes first. The rules of IDEA for each state (ectacenter.org/sec619/stateregs.asp) are available from the Early Childhood Technical Assistance (ECTA) Center.

The IDEA requires that children be taught in the least restrictive environment appropriate for them. This means the teaching environment should meet a child's needs and skills while minimizing restrictions to typical learning experiences.

Individualized Education Programs

Children who qualify for special education services will receive an Individualized Education Program, or IEP. This personalized and written education plan:

- Lists goals for the child
- Specifies the services the child will receive
- Lists the specialists who will work with the child

Qualifying for Special Education

To qualify for special education services, a child must be evaluated by the school system and meet federal and state guidelines. Parents and caregivers can contact their school principal or special education coordinator to find out how to have their child evaluated. Parents can also review these resources:

- The Center for Parent Information and Resources (www.parentcenterhub. org) offers information about Parent Training and Information Centers and Community Parent Resource Centers (www.parentcenterhub.org/ the-parent-center-network).
- IDEA Parent Guide (www.ncld.org/get-involved/learn-the-law/ idea-parent-guide)

Interventions for Specific Learning Disabilities

Below are just a few of the ways schools help children with specific learning disabilities.

Dyslexia

- **Intensive teaching techniques.** These can include specific, step-by-step, and very methodical approaches to teaching reading with the goal of improving both spoken language and written language skills. These techniques are generally more intensive in terms of how often they occur and how long they last and often involve small group or one-on-one instruction.
- **Classroom modifications.** Teachers can give students with dyslexia extra time to finish tasks and provide taped tests that allow the child to hear the questions instead of reading them.
- **Use of technology.** Children with dyslexia may benefit from listening to audiobooks or using word-processing programs.

Dysgraphia

- **Special tools.** Teachers can offer oral exams, provide a note-taker, or allow the child to videotape reports instead of writing them. Computer software can facilitate children being able to produce written text.
- **Use of technology.** A child with dysgraphia can be taught to use word-processing programs, including those incorporating speech-to-text translation, or an audio recorder instead of writing by hand.

- **Reducing the need for writing.** Teachers can provide notes, outlines, and preprinted study sheets.

Dyscalculia
- **Visual techniques.** Teachers can draw pictures of word problems and show the student how to use colored pencils to differentiate parts of problems.
- **Memory aids.** Rhymes and music can help a child remember math concepts.
- **Computers.** A child with dyscalculia can use a computer for drills and practice.

Tips for Managing a Learning Disability in Adulthood
Support from schools can improve elementary and secondary students' math, reading, and other language skills. But, how can people with learning disabilities prepare for the demands of university or working life?

Be Your Own Advocate
It is important to know and speak up for what you need. Understand your learning challenges, identify possible solutions, and ask for the resources that will allow you to reach your goals.

Ensure That Your Surroundings Facilitate Success
Work with your school or employer to create a supportive learning environment, such as access to software that will help you succeed now and in the future.

Take Advantage of Assistive Technology
Use computer tools customized to your own pace and needs that can read text aloud, help you articulate your thoughts, and provide structure to your writing.

CHAPTER 10
CONDITIONS RELATED TO LEARNING DISABILITIES

About This Chapter: Text in this chapter begins with excerpts from "What Conditions Are Related to Learning Disabilities?" *Eunice Kennedy Shriver* National Institute of Child Health and Human Development (NICHD), September 11, 2018; Text under the heading "Developmental Disabilities" is excerpted from "Facts about Developmental Disabilities," Centers for Disease Control and Prevention (CDC), September 26, 2019.

Children with learning disabilities may be at greater risk for certain conditions compared to other kids. Recognizing and treating these conditions can help a child be more successful.

Attention Deficit Hyperactivity Disorder

Attention deficit hyperactivity disorder (ADHD) occurs more frequently in children with learning disabilities compared to children without learning disabilities. A child with a learning disability who also has ADHD may be distracted easily and find it harder to concentrate.

A *Eunice Kennedy Shriver* National Institute of Child Health and Human Development (NICHD) supported study on reading disorders found that it is important to treat both the ADHD symptoms and reading problems. The findings show that although both disorders need separate treatments, these interventions can be done effectively at the same time.

Depression/Anxiety

A child with a learning disability may struggle with low self-esteem, frustration, worry, and other problems. Mental-health professionals can help the child understand these feelings, learn ways to cope with them, and learn how to build healthy relationships.

Developmental Disabilities

Developmental disabilities begin anytime during the developmental period and usually last throughout a person's lifetime. Most developmental disabilities begin before a baby is born, but some can happen after birth because of injury, infection, or other factors.

Most developmental disabilities are thought to be caused by a complex mix of factors. These factors include genetics; parental health and behaviors (such as smoking and drinking) during pregnancy; complications during birth; infections the mother might have during pregnancy or the baby might have very early in life; and exposure of the mother or child to high levels of environmental toxins, such as lead. For some developmental disabilities, such as fetal alcohol syndrome, which is caused by drinking alcohol during pregnancy, we know the cause. But for most, we do not.

Following are some examples of what we know about specific developmental disabilities:

- At least 25 percent of hearing loss among babies is due to maternal infections during pregnancy, such as cytomegalovirus (CMV) infection; complications after birth; and head trauma.
- Some of the most common known causes of intellectual disability include fetal alcohol syndrome; genetic and chromosomal conditions, such as Down syndrome and fragile X syndrome (FXS); and certain infections during pregnancy.
- Children who have a sibling with autism are at a higher risk of also having autism spectrum disorder (ASD).
- Low birth weight, premature birth, multiple birth, and infections during pregnancy are associated with an increased risk for many developmental disabilities.
- Untreated newborn jaundice (high levels of bilirubin in the blood during the first few days after birth) can cause a type of brain damage known as "kernicterus." Children with kernicterus are more likely to have cerebral palsy, hearing and vision problems, and problems with their teeth. Early detection and treatment of newborn jaundice can prevent kernicterus.

CHAPTER 11
STATISTICS ON LEARNING DISABILITIES

About This Chapter: This chapter includes text excerpted from "Students with Disabilities," U.S. Department of Education (ED), May 2020.

Students with Disabilities

In 2018–19, the number of students ages 3 to 21 who received special education services under the Individuals with Disabilities Education Act (IDEA) was 7.1 million, or 14 percent of all public-school students. Among students receiving special education services, 33 percent had specific learning disabilities.

Enacted in 1975, the IDEA formerly known as the "Education for All Handicapped Children Act," mandates the provision of a free and appropriate public-school education for eligible students ages 3 to 21. Eligible students are those identified by a team of professionals as having a disability that adversely affects academic performance and as being in need of special education and related services. Data collection activities to monitor compliance with IDEA began in 1976.

From school year 2000–01 through 2004–05, the number of students ages 3 to 21 who received special education services under IDEA increased from 6.3 million, or 13 percent of total public school enrollment, to 6.7 million, or 14 percent of total public school enrollment. Both the number and the percentage of students served under IDEA declined from 2004–05 through 2011–12. Between 2011–12 and 2018–19, the number of students served increased from 6.4 million to 7.1 million and the percentage served increased from 13 percent of total public school enrollment to 14 percent of total public school enrollment.

The Individuals with Disabilities Education Act (IDEA), by Disability Type: School Year 2018–19

In the school year 2018–19, a higher percentage of students ages 3 to 21 received special education services under IDEA for specific learning disabilities than for any other type of disability. A specific learning disability is a disorder in one or more of the basic psychological processes involved in understanding or using language, spoken

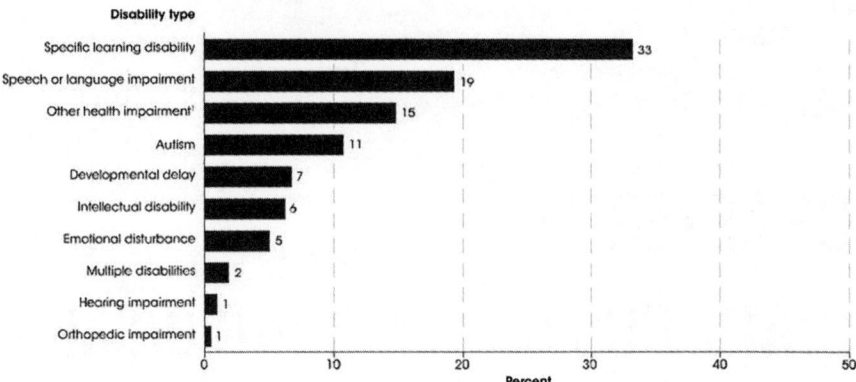

Disability type

Figure 11.1. Percentage Distribution of Students Ages 3 to 21 *(Source: U.S. Department of Education (ED), Office of Special Education Programs (OSEP), Individuals with Disabilities Education Act (IDEA) database)*

[1]Other health impairments include having limited strength, vitality, or alertness due to chronic or acute health problems such as a heart condition, tuberculosis, rheumatic fever, nephritis, asthma, sickle cell anemia, hemophilia, epilepsy, lead poisoning, leukemia, or diabetes.
NOTE: Data are for the 50 states and the District of Columbia (DC) only. Includes 2015–16 data for 3- to 21-year-olds in Wisconsin due to unavailability of more recent data for children served in Wisconsin. Visual impairment, traumatic brain injury, and deaf-blindness are not shown because they each account for less than 0.5 percent of students served under IDEA. Due to categories not shown, detail does not sum to 100 percent. Although rounded numbers are displayed, the figures are based on unrounded data.

or written, that may manifest itself in an imperfect ability to listen, think, speak, read, write, spell, or do mathematical calculations. In 2018–19, some 33 percent of all students who received special education services had specific learning disabilities, 19 percent had speech or language impairments, and 15 percent had other health impairments (including having limited strength, vitality, or alertness due to chronic or acute health problems such as a heart condition, tuberculosis, rheumatic fever, nephritis, asthma, sickle cell anemia, hemophilia, epilepsy, lead poisoning, leukemia, or diabetes). Students with autism, developmental delays, intellectual disabilities, and emotional disturbances each accounted for between 5 and 11 percent of students served under IDEA. Students with multiple disabilities, hearing impairments, orthopedic impairments, visual impairments, traumatic brain injuries, and deaf-blindness each accounted for two percent or less of those served under IDEA.

The Individuals with Disabilities Education Act (IDEA), by Race/Ethnicity: School Year 2018–19

In the school year 2018–19, the percentage (out of total public school enrollment) of students ages 3 to 21 who received special education services under IDEA differed by race/ethnicity. The percentage of students served under IDEA was highest for American

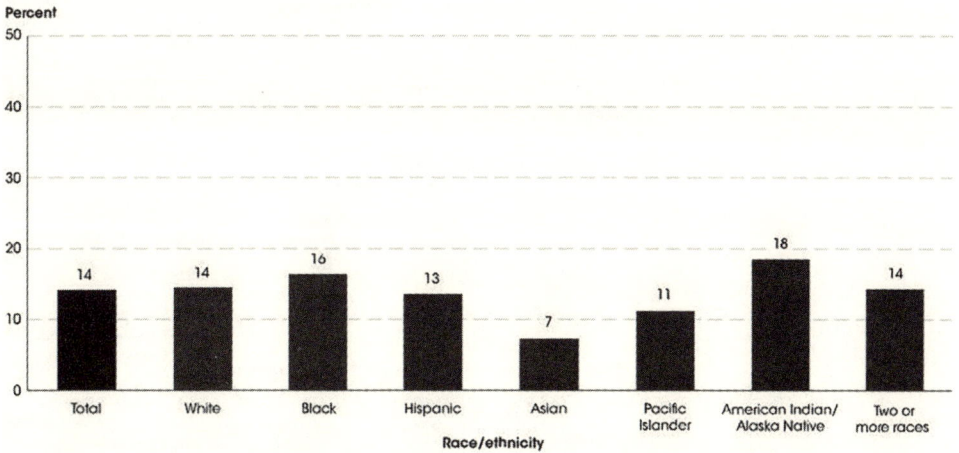

Percent

Figure 11.2. Percentage of Students Ages 3 to 21 *(Source: U.S. Department of Education (ED), Office of Special Education Programs (OSEP), Individuals with Disabilities Education Act (IDEA) database)*

NOTE: *Based on the total public school enrollment in prekindergarten through grade 12 by race/ ethnicity. Although data are for the 50 states and the DC, data limitations result in inclusion of a small (but unknown) number of students from other jurisdictions. Includes 2015–16 data for 3- to 21-year-olds in Wisconsin due to unavailability of more recent data for children served in Wisconsin. Race categories exclude persons of Hispanic ethnicity. Although rounded numbers are displayed, the figures are based on unrounded data.*

Indian/Alaska Native students (18%), followed by black students (16%), white students and students of two or more races (14% each), Hispanic students (13%), Pacific Islander students (11%), and Asian students (7%).

Among Hispanic, American Indian/Alaska Native, Pacific Islander, and white students ages 3 to 21, the percentage of students who received special education services in 2018–19 for specific learning disabilities combined with the percentage who received services for speech or language impairments accounted for 50 percent or more of students served under IDEA. Among their peers who were black, of two or more races, and Asian, the percentage accounted for between 40 and 50 percent of students served under IDEA. The percentage distribution of various types of special education services received by students differed by race/ethnicity. For example, the percentage of students with disabilities who received services under IDEA for specific learning disabilities was lower for Asian students (19%), students of two or more races (29%), and white students (29%) than for students overall (33%). However, the percentage of students with disabilities who received services under IDEA for autism was higher for Asian students (25%) and students of two or more races (12%) than for students overall (11%). Additionally, among students served under IDEA, seven percent each of black students and students of two or more races received services for

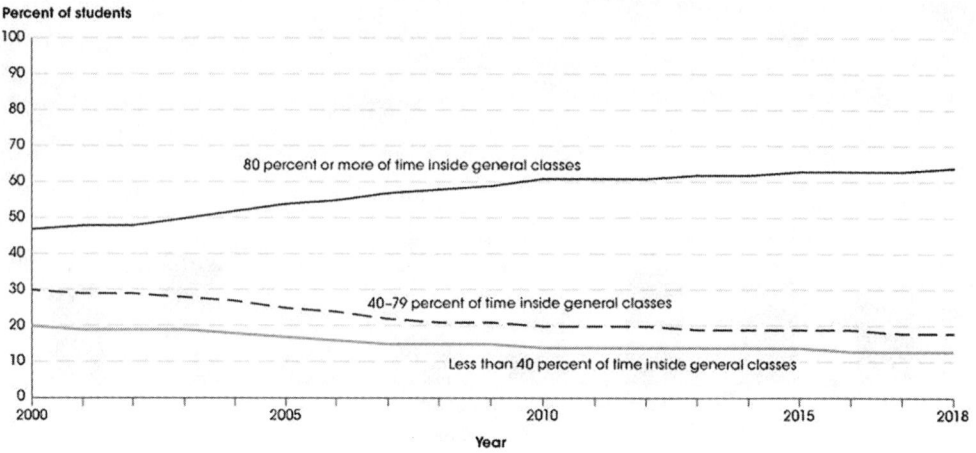

Figure 11.3. Among Students Ages 6 to 21 *(Source: U.S. Department of Education (ED), Office of Special Education Programs (OSEP), Individuals with Disabilities Education Act (IDEA) database)*

NOTE: Data are for the 50 states and the DC only. Fall 2016, 2017, and 2018 include fall 2015 data for 6- to 21-year-olds in Wisconsin due to unavailability of fall 2016, 2017, and 2018 data for children served in Wisconsin. Fall 2017 also includes fall 2016 data for 6- to 21-year-olds in Maine and Vermont due to unavailability of fall 2017 data for children in that age group served in those states.

emotional disturbances. In comparison, five percent of all students served under IDEA received services for emotional disturbances.

Separate data on special education services for males and females are available only for students ages 6 to 21, rather than ages 3 to 21. Among those 6- to 21-year-old students enrolled in public schools in 2018–19, a higher percentage of male students (18%) than of female students (10%) received special education services under IDEA. In addition, the percentage distribution of 6- to 21-year-old students who received various types of special education services in 2018–19 differed by sex. For example, the percentage of students served under IDEA who received services for specific learning disabilities was higher for female students (44%) than for male students (34%), while the percentage served under IDEA who received services for autism was higher for male students (13%) than for female students (5%).

The Individuals with Disabilities Education Act (IDEA), Percentage Who Spent Various Amounts of Time inside General Classes: Fall 2000 through Fall 2018

Educational environment data are also available for students ages 6 to 21 served under IDEA. About 95 percent of students ages 6 to 21 served under IDEA in fall 2018 were enrolled in regular schools. Three percent of students served under IDEA were enrolled in separate schools (public or private) for students with disabilities; one percent were placed by their parents in regular private schools; and less than one percent each were home bound or in hospitals, in separate residential facilities (public or private), or in correctional facilities. Among all students ages 6 to 21 served under IDEA, the percentage who spent most of the school day (i.e., 80% or more of their time) inside general classes in regular schools increased from 47 percent in fall 2000 to 64 percent in fall 2018. In contrast, during the same period, the percentage of students who spent 40 to 79 percent of the school day inside general classes decreased from 30 to 18 percent, and the percentage of students who spent less than 40 percent of their time inside general classes decreased from 20 to 13 percent. In fall 2018, the percentage of students served under IDEA who spent most of the school day inside general classes was highest for students with speech or language impairments (88%). Approximately two-thirds of students with specific learning disabilities (72%), visual impairments (68%), other health impairments (67%), developmental delays (66%), and hearing impairments (63%) spent most of the school day inside general classes. In contrast, 17 percent of students with intellectual disabilities and 14 percent of students with multiple disabilities spent most of the school day inside general classes.

Data are also available for students ages 14 to 21 served under IDEA who exited school during the school year 2017–18, including exit reason. Approximately 414,000 students ages 14 to 21 served under IDEA exited school in 2017–18: over two-thirds (73%) graduated with a regular high school diploma, 16 percent dropped out, 10 percent received an alternative certificate, one percent reached the maximum age 6 to receive special education services, and less than one-half of one percent died.

The Individuals with Disabilities Education Act (IDEA) Who Exited School, Percentage Who Exited for Selected Reasons, by Race/Ethnicity: School Year 2017–18

Among students ages 14 to 21 served under IDEA who exited school in the school year 2017–18, the percentages who graduated with a regular high school diploma, received an alternative certificate, and dropped out differed by race/ethnicity. The percentage of exiting students who graduated with a regular high school diploma was highest for Asian students (79%) and lowest for black students (66%). The percentage of exiting students who received an alternative certificate was highest for black students (12%) and lowest for American Indian/Alaska Native students (4%). The percentage of exiting students who dropped out in 2017–18 was highest for American Indian/Alaska Native students (24%) and lowest for Asian students (7%).

Among students ages 14 to 21 served under IDEA who exited school in school year 2017–18, the percentages who graduated with a regular high school diploma, received an alternative certificate, and dropped out also differed by type of disability. The percentage of exiting students who graduated with a regular high school diploma was highest for students with speech or language impairments (86%) and lowest for students with multiple disabilities (47%). The percentage of exiting students who

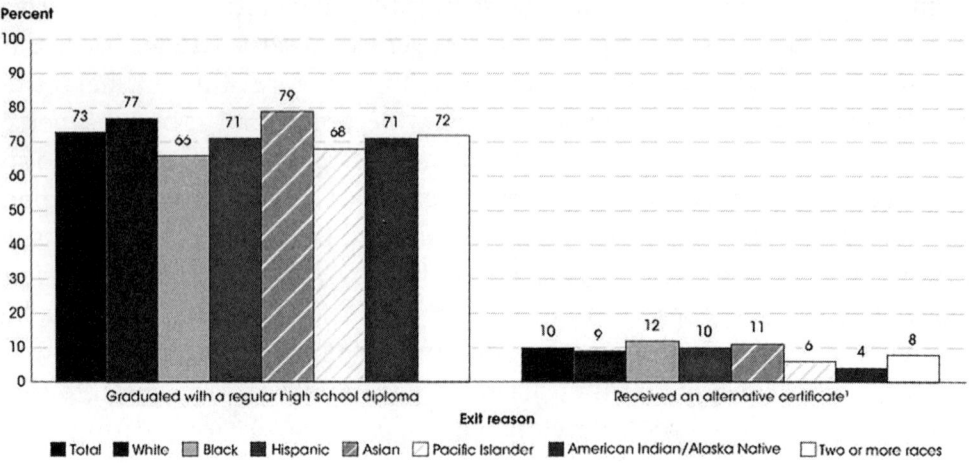

Percent

Figure 11.4. Among Students Ages 14 to 21 *(Source: U.S. Department of Education (ED), Office of Special Education Programs (OSEP), Individuals with Disabilities Education Act (IDEA) database)*

[1]Received a certificate of completion, modified diploma, or some similar document, but did not meet the same standards for graduation as those for students without disabilities.
NOTE: Data in this figure are for the 50 states, the DC, the Bureau of Indian Education, American Samoa, the Federated States of Micronesia, Guam, the Northern Marianas, Puerto Rico, the Republic of Palau, the Republic of the Marshall Islands, and the U.S. Virgin Islands. Data for all other figures in this indicator are for the 50 states and the DC only. Includes imputations for missing or unavailable data from Vermont. Race categories exclude persons of Hispanic ethnicity. Although rounded numbers are displayed, the figures are based on unrounded data.

received an alternative certificate was highest for students with intellectual disabilities (32%) and lowest for students with speech or language impairments (3%). The percentage of exiting students who dropped out in 2017–18 was highest for students with emotional disturbances (32%) and lowest for students with deaf-blindness (5%).

CHAPTER 12
NICHD LEARNING DISABILITIES RESEARCH

About This Chapter: This chapter includes text excerpted from "NICHD Learning Disabilities Research Information," *Eunice Kennedy Shriver* National Institute of Child Health and Human Development (NICHD), September 11, 2018.

The *Eunice Kennedy Shriver* National Institute of Child Health and Human Development (NICHD) is one of several federal agencies that support and conduct research on learning disabilities and disorders. The institute's research portfolio includes studies investigating the causes, development, neurobiology, prevention, and remediation of learning disabilities. In addition, the NICHD provides funding to train researchers in this field.

The *Eunice Kennedy Shriver* National Institute of Child Health and Human Development Research Goals

The NICHD aims to prevent learning disabilities when possible and to intervene early when learning difficulties or disabilities and associated conditions occur through two programs: the Reading, Writing, and Related Learning Disabilities (RWRLD) program (www.nichd.nih.gov/about/org/der/branches/cdbb/programs#reading) and the Mathematics and Science Cognition, Reasoning, and Learning (MSCRL): Development and Disorders program (www.nichd.nih.gov/about/org/der/branches/cdbb/programs#mathematics).

The NICHD research goals related to learning disabilities include:
- Understanding the role of the individual's environment, their genes, their brain, their behavior, and their thinking and memory processes
- Investigating the genetic and neurobiological foundations of these disabilities
- Creating measurement tools to identify children at risk
- Developing and evaluating prevention methods
- Developing and assessing remediation and instructional approaches that promote learning

Research Activities and Advances

Learning disabilities can take a toll on children and their families. The NICHD supports research to address reading, writing, math, and related disabilities and disorders.

Institute Activities and Advances

The NICHD has a history of supporting research on learning disabilities and related conditions. The Child Development and Behavior Branch (CDBB) supports much of the research in this area through the Reading, Writing, and Related Learning Disabilities program (www.nichd.nih.gov/about/org/der/branches/cdbb/programs#reading) and the Mathematics and Science Cognition, Reasoning, and Learning: Development and Disorders program (www.nichd.nih.gov/about/org/der/branches/cdbb/programs#mathematics).

The RWRLD program focuses on research and training to understand how reading and writing skills develop during a person's life. One goal is to develop ways to prevent these disabilities. Another goal is to develop better teaching methods for reading and writing skills. The program includes studies to integrate what you learn about the genetic, neurobiological, and cognitive/behavioral causes. It includes studies on ways to help children with reading and writing disabilities. The program also includes studies to develop measurement tools to support these efforts. RWRLD's efforts are complemented by other CDBB programs. These include the Early Learning and School Readiness program (www.nichd.nih.gov/about/org/der/branches/cdbb/programs#early-learning); the Language, Bilingualism, and Biliteracy program (www.nichd.nih.gov/about/org/der/branches/cdbb/programs#language); and the Behavioral Pediatrics and Health Promotion Research program (www.nichd.nih.gov/about/org/der/branches/cdbb/programs#behavioral).

The MSCRL focuses on research on mathematical thinking and problem-solving. The program funds research on scientific reasoning, learning, and discovery from infancy to early adulthood. It explores factors that may contribute to atypical development in mathematics and science learning and thinking. These influences include genetic and neurobiological factors. They also include cognitive, language, sociocultural, and instructional factors. This research also:

- Investigates individual differences that affect achievement in math and science
- Delineates the skills needed to improve in these areas
- Develops ways to address learning difficulties that frequently emerge in math and science
- Develops instructional methods to reduce these learning difficulties

In 1997, the NICHD and the U.S. Department of Education (ED) created the National Reading Panel (www.nichd.nih.gov/research/supported/nrp) to draw on scientific evidence to identify the best ways to teach children to read. The Panel's report (www.nichd.nih.gov/publications/product/64?pubs_id=89), which included research supported by the RWRLD program, noted that children who received explicit instruction in specific components of reading were more successful readers than those who did not receive such instruction. The Panel's findings have since contributed to nationwide standards in education.

The NICHD-sponsored research also influenced the 2004 revision of the IDEA legislation. The research demonstrated the limitations of identifying reading disabilities based solely on discrepancies between a child's IQ and achievement. This is called the "discrepancy model." Now, states can consider alternative approaches to identifying learning disabilities, and educators can provide early intervention.

In a related study, the NICHD-sponsored researchers used brain imaging technology to compare the brain functioning of poor readers with low IQ scores and poor readers with typical IQ scores. They found no reliable functional brain differences between the two groups, thereby strengthening the evidence against the discrepancy model.

Improvements in brain imaging technology have helped researchers understand learning disabilities much better. For example, the NICHD-supported researchers used brain imaging to show that the functional brain patterns of poor readers change with successful reading remediation to more closely resemble that of skilled readers.

Researchers also are looking at how genes interact with each other and with the environment to increase the risk for learning disabilities. The goal is to better understand what causes or affects learning disabilities and create interventions. For example, the NICHD-supported researchers found a dyslexia-susceptibility gene and helped find how it links to reading ability. Using long-term studies of twins, another NICHD-supported study showed that genes' effects on reading performance are also affected by a child's environment.

The NICHD-funded researchers are also working to understand dyscalculia. One study found that people with dyscalculia may have difficulty understanding that any number or quantity can be broken into smaller numbers. The study also found that children considered low achievers who do not have dyscalculia struggle less with math than children with the disorder. In part, this is because children without dyscalculia are better able to memorize new math facts. Another study found that having a less sensitive ability to estimate and compare quantities without counting may underlie dyscalculia. In children without dyscalculia but with low math achievement scores, this ability appeared similar to that of their typically achieving peers. This suggests that children with dyscalculia have different deficits and need interventions designed to target these unique challenges.

Other Activities and Advances

The NICHD continues to create, collaborate in, and support activities to advance the field. These efforts include the following:

- Staff at the CDBB collaborated with the former National Institute for Literacy (NIFL) to develop and revise a number of NIFL publications, including Put Reading First: The Research Building Blocks for Teaching Children to Read (www.nichd.nih.gov/publications/product/239?pubs_id=226), a resource on evidence-based instruction for teachers, as well as reading publications for parents and families (www.nichd.nih.gov/publications/list/collection?g=7&col=18&cat=all).
- The NICHD's Learning Disabilities Research Centers Consortium (www.nichd.nih.gov/research/supported/ldrc) investigates the causes, origins, and development of learning disabilities. The consortium is identifying the genetic, brain-related, and treatment characteristics of children, adolescents, and adults with learning disabilities.
- The NICHD supported the National Early Literacy Panel (NELP) (lincs.ed.gov/earlychildhood/NELP/NELP09.html), which convened in 2002 to review research on the development of early literacy skills in children ages 0 to 5. The aim was to identify the early skills that are important to literacy, to identify the teaching methods that teachers and parents could use to support those early skills, and to contribute to the educational policies that will enhance literacy. This effort resulted in the Developing Early Literacy: Executive Summary of the NELP (www.nichd.nih.gov/publications/product/345?pubs_id=574) and the Developing Early Literacy: Report of the NELP (www.nichd.nih.gov/publications/product/346?pubs_id=5750) publications.
- Developing Literacy in Second-Language Learners (www.cal.org/resource-center/publications-products/developing-literacy), the report of the National Literacy Panel on Children and Youth, was partially funded by the NICHD along with the ED. This report includes research supported by the NICHD on bilingualism, second-language learning, and cross-linguistic studies of reading.

PART 2 | TYPES OF LEARNING DISABILITIES

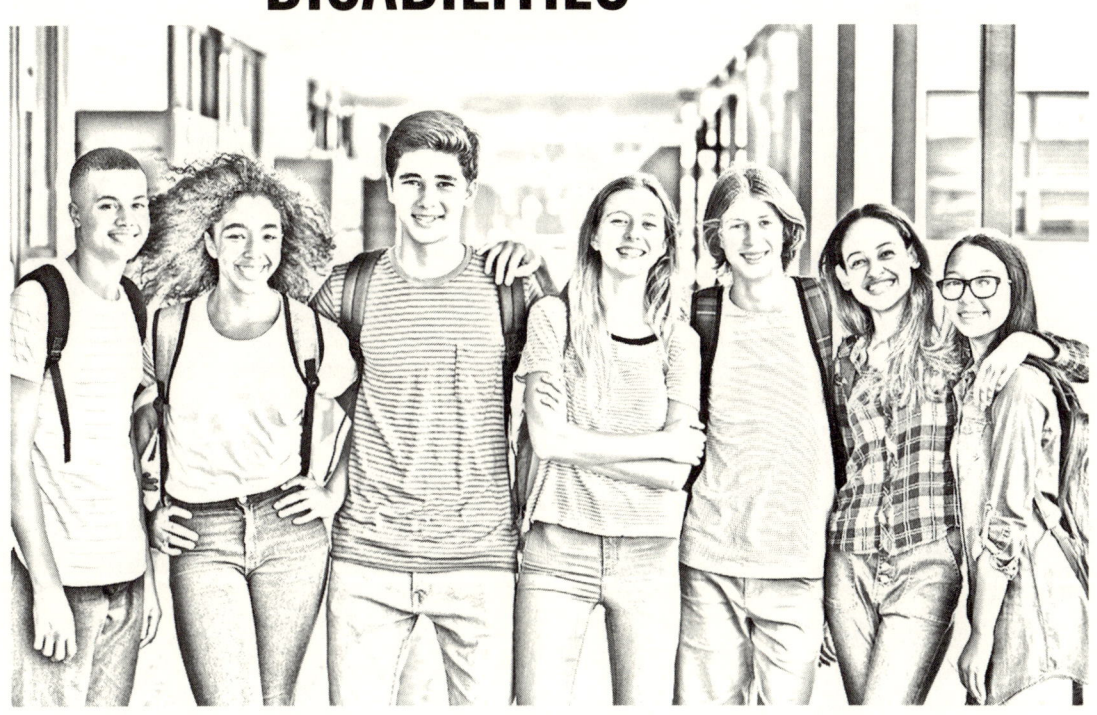

CHAPTER 13
ATTENTION DEFICIT HYPERACTIVITY DISORDER

About This Chapter: This chapter includes text excerpted from "Attention Deficit Hyperactivity Disorder," National Institute of Mental Health (NIMH), September 2019.

What Is Attention Deficit Hyperactivity Disorder?

Attention deficit hyperactivity disorder (ADHD) is a disorder marked by an ongoing pattern of inattention and/or hyperactivity-impulsivity that interferes with functioning or development.

- **Inattention** means a person wanders off task, lacks persistence, has difficulty sustaining focus, and is disorganized; and these problems are not due to defiance or lack of comprehension.
- **Hyperactivity** means a person seems to move about constantly, including in situations in which it is not appropriate; or excessively fidgets, taps, or talks. In adults, it may be extreme restlessness or wearing others out with constant activity.
- **Impulsivity** means a person makes hasty actions that occur in the moment without first thinking about them and that may have a high potential for harm, or a desire for immediate rewards or inability to delay gratification. An impulsive person may be socially intrusive and excessively interrupt others or make important decisions without considering the long-term consequences.

Signs and Symptoms of Attention Deficit Hyperactivity Disorder

Inattention and hyperactivity/impulsivity are the key behaviors of ADHD. Some people with ADHD only have problems with one of the behaviors, while others have both inattention and hyperactivity-impulsivity. Most children have the combined type of ADHD.

In preschool, the most common ADHD symptom is hyperactivity.

It is normal to have some inattention, unfocused motor activity, and impulsivity, but for people with ADHD, these behaviors:

- Are more severe
- Occur more often
- Interfere with or reduce the quality of how they function socially, at school, or in a job

Inattention

People with symptoms of inattention may often:

- Overlook or miss details, make careless mistakes in schoolwork, at work, or during other activities
- Have problems sustaining attention in tasks or play, including conversations, lectures, or lengthy reading
- Not seem to listen when spoken to directly
- Not follow through on instructions and fail to finish schoolwork, chores, or duties in the workplace or start tasks but quickly lose focus and get easily sidetracked
- Have problems organizing tasks and activities, such as what to do in sequence, keeping materials and belongings in order, having messy work and poor time management, and failing to meet deadlines
- Avoid or dislike tasks that require sustained mental effort, such as schoolwork or homework, or for teens and older adults, preparing reports, completing forms, or reviewing lengthy papers
- Lose things necessary for tasks or activities, such as school supplies, pencils, books, tools, wallets, keys, paperwork, eyeglasses, and cell phones
- Be easily distracted by unrelated thoughts or stimuli
- Be forgetful in daily activities, such as chores, errands, returning calls, and keeping appointments

Hyperactivity-Impulsivity

People with symptoms of hyperactivity-impulsivity may often:

- Fidget and squirm in their seats
- Leave their seats in situations when staying seated is expected, such as in the classroom or the office
- Run or dash around or climb in situations where it is inappropriate or, in teens and adults, often feel restless
- Be unable to play or engage in hobbies quietly
- Be constantly in motion or "on the go," or act as if "driven by a motor"
- Talk nonstop

- Blurt out an answer before a question has been completed, finish other people's sentences, or speak without waiting for a turn in a conversation
- Have trouble waiting for her or his turn
- Interrupt or intrude on others, for example in conversations, games, or activities

Diagnosis of ADHD requires a comprehensive evaluation by a licensed clinician, such as a pediatrician, psychologist, or psychiatrist with expertise in ADHD. For a person to receive a diagnosis of ADHD, the symptoms of inattention and/or hyperactivity-impulsivity must be chronic or long-lasting, impair the person's functioning, and cause the person to fall behind typical development for her or his age. The doctor will also ensure that any ADHD symptoms are not due to another medical or psychiatric condition. Most children with ADHD receive a diagnosis during the elementary school years. For an adolescent or adult to receive a diagnosis of ADHD, the symptoms need to have been present before age 12.

Attention deficit hyperactivity disorder symptoms can appear as early as between the ages of 3 and 6 and can continue through adolescence and adulthood. Symptoms of ADHD can be mistaken for emotional or disciplinary problems or missed entirely in quiet, well-behaved children, leading to a delay in diagnosis. Adults with undiagnosed ADHD may have a history of poor academic performance, problems at work, or difficult or failed relationships.

Attention deficit hyperactivity disorder symptoms can change over time as a person ages. In young children with ADHD, hyperactivity-impulsivity is the most predominant symptom. As a child reaches elementary school, the symptom of inattention may become more prominent and cause the child to struggle academically. In adolescence, hyperactivity seems to lessen and may show more often as feelings of restlessness or fidgeting, but inattention and impulsivity may remain. Many adolescents with ADHD also struggle with relationships and antisocial behaviors. Inattention, restlessness, and impulsivity tend to persist into adulthood.

Risk Factors of Attention Deficit Hyperactivity Disorder

Researchers are not sure what causes ADHD. Like many other illnesses, several factors can contribute to ADHD, such as:
- Genes
- Cigarette smoking, alcohol use, or drug use during pregnancy
- Exposure to environmental toxins during pregnancy
- Exposure to environmental toxins, such as high levels of lead, at a young age
- Low birth weight
- Brain injuries

Attention deficit hyperactivity disorder is more common in males than females, and females with ADHD are more likely to have problems primarily with inattention. Other conditions, such as learning disabilities, anxiety disorder, conduct disorder, depression, and substance abuse, are common in people with ADHD.

Treatment and Therapies of Attention Deficit Hyperactivity Disorder

While there is no cure for ADHD, currently available treatments can help reduce symptoms and improve functioning. Treatments include medication, psychotherapy, education or training, or a combination of treatments.

Medication

For many people, ADHD medications reduce hyperactivity and impulsivity and improve their ability to focus, work, and learn. Medication also may improve physical coordination. Sometimes several different medications or dosages must be tried before finding the right one that works for a particular person. Anyone taking medications must be monitored closely and carefully by their prescribing doctor.

Stimulants. The most common type of medication used for treating ADHD is called a "stimulant." Although it may seem unusual to treat ADHD with a medication that is considered a stimulant, it works by increasing the brain chemicals dopamine and norepinephrine, which play essential roles in thinking and attention.

Under medical supervision, stimulant medications are considered safe. However, there are risks and side effects, especially when misused or taken in excess of the prescribed dose. For example, stimulants can raise blood pressure and heart rate and increase anxiety. Therefore, a person with other health problems, including high blood pressure, seizures, heart disease, glaucoma, liver or kidney disease, or an anxiety disorder should tell their doctor before taking a stimulant.

Talk with a doctor if you see any of these or other side effects while taking stimulants:

- Decreased appetite
- Sleep problems
- Tics (sudden, repetitive movements or sounds)
- Personality changes
- Increased anxiety and irritability
- Stomachaches
- Headaches

Nonstimulants. A few other ADHD medications are nonstimulants. These medications take longer to start working than stimulants, but can also improve focus, attention, and impulsivity in a person with ADHD. Doctors may prescribe a nonstimulant: when a person has bothersome side effects from stimulants; when a stimulant was not effective; or in combination with a stimulant to increase effectiveness.

Although not approved by the U.S. Food and Drug Administration (FDA) specifically for the treatment of ADHD, some antidepressants are sometimes used alone or in combination with a stimulant to treat ADHD. Antidepressants may help all of the symptoms of ADHD and can be prescribed if a patient has bothersome side effects from stimulants. Antidepressants can be helpful in combination with stimulants if a patient also has another condition, such as an anxiety disorder, depression, or another mood disorder.

Psychotherapy and Psychosocial Interventions

Several specific psychosocial interventions have been shown to help patients and their families manage symptoms and improve everyday functioning. In addition, children and adults with ADHD need guidance and understanding from their parents, families, and teachers to reach their full potential and to succeed.

For school-age children, frustration, blame, and anger may have built up within a family before a child is diagnosed. Parents and children may need specialized help to overcome negative feelings. Mental-health professionals can educate parents about ADHD and how it affects a family. They also will help the child and her or his parents develop new skills, attitudes, and ways of relating to each other.

Behavioral therapy is a type of psychotherapy that aims to help a person change her or his behavior. It might involve practical assistance, such as help organizing tasks or completing schoolwork, or working through emotionally difficult events. Behavioral therapy also teaches a person how to:

- Monitor her or his own behavior
- Give oneself praise or rewards for acting in a desired way, such as controlling anger or thinking before acting

Parents, teachers, and family members also can give positive or negative feedback for certain behaviors and help establish clear rules, chore lists, and other structured routines to help a person control her or his behavior. Therapists may also teach children social skills, such as how to wait their turn, share toys, ask for help, or respond to teasing. Learning to read facial expressions and the tone of voice in others, and how to respond appropriately can also be part of social skills training.

Cognitive-behavioral therapy (CBT) can also teach a person mindfulness techniques, or meditation. A person learns how to be aware and accepting of one's own thoughts and feelings to improve focus and concentration. The therapist also encourages the person with ADHD to adjust to the life changes that come with treatment, such as thinking before acting, or resisting the urge to take unnecessary risks.

Tips to Help Kids with ADHD Stay Organized

Parents and teachers can help kids with ADHD stay organized and follow directions with tools such as:

- **Keeping a routine and a schedule.** Keep the same routine every day, from wake-up time to bedtime. Include times for homework, outdoor play, and indoor activities. Keep the schedule on the refrigerator or a bulletin board in the kitchen. Write changes on the schedule as far in advance as possible.
- **Organizing everyday items.** Have a place for everything, (such as clothing, backpacks, and toys), and keep everything in its place.
- **Using homework and notebook organizers.** Use organizers for school material and supplies. Stress to your child the importance of writing down assignments and bringing home the necessary books.
- **Being clear and consistent.** Children with ADHD need consistent rules they can understand and follow.
- **Giving praise or rewards when rules are followed.** Children with ADHD often receive and expect criticism. Look for good behavior and praise it.

Family and marital therapy can help family members and spouses find better ways to handle disruptive behaviors, to encourage behavior changes, and improve interactions with the patient.

Parenting skills training (behavioral parent management training) teaches parents the skills they need to encourage and reward positive behaviors in their children. It helps parents learn how to use a system of rewards and consequences to change a child's behavior. Parents are taught to give immediate and positive feedback for behaviors they want to encourage and ignore or redirect behaviors that they want to discourage. They may also learn to structure situations in ways that support desired behavior.

Specific behavioral classroom management interventions have been shown to be effective for managing youths' symptoms and improving their functioning at school and with peers. These research-informed strategies typically include teacher-implemented reward programs that often utilize point systems and communication with parents via Daily Report Cards.

Many schools offer special education services to children with ADHD who qualify. Educational specialists help the child, parents, and teachers make changes to classroom and homework assignments to help the child succeed. Public schools are required to offer these services for qualified children, which may be free for families living within the school district.

Stress-management techniques can benefit parents of children with ADHD by increasing their ability to deal with frustration so that they can respond calmly to their child's behavior.

Support groups can help parents and families connect with others who have similar problems and concerns. Groups often meet regularly to share frustrations and successes, to exchange information about recommended specialists and strategies, and to talk with experts.

CHAPTER 14
DYSCALCULIA: MATH DISABILITY

About This Chapter: Text beginning with the heading "What Is Dyscalculia?" is excerpted from "Infographic: Does Your Child Struggle with Math?" *Eunice Kennedy Shriver* National Institute of Child Health and Human Development (NICHD), December 30, 2017; Text beginning with the heading "Symptoms of Dyscalculia" is © 2017 Omnigraphics. Reviewed July 2020.

What Is Dyscalculia?
Dyscalculia is not as well-known as dyslexia, but both are learning disabilities.

Dyscalculia = Math
Causes trouble with:
- Understanding arithmetic (numbers) concepts and solving arithmetic problems
- Estimating time, measuring, and budgeting

It is also called a "**math learning disability.**"

How Many People Have Dyscalculia?
- More than 20 million people
- Boys are slightly more likely to have dyscalculia than girls

What Are the Risk Factors for Dyscalculia?
By Age 4
Has trouble:
- Listing numbers in correct order
- Matching number words or written digits to number of objects
- Counting objects

Age 6 to 12

Has regular and lasting trouble:
- Performing addition, subtraction, multiplication, or division appropriate to grade level
- Recognizing math errors

Age 12+

Has trouble:
- Estimating (informed guessing)
- Making exact calculations
- Understanding graphs and charts
- Understanding fractions and decimals

How Can Adults Reduce the Risk of Dyscalculia in Young Children?

Show the child that numbers are a normal part of everyday life.
- Mention numbers to your child while doing everyday activities—like grocery shopping or setting the table
- Count out loud and show the child both the written number word ("three") and digit ("3")
- Count actual objects the child can see
- Compare objects in everyday conversation using words that describe size or amount

Symptoms of Dyscalculia

In early childhood, dyscalculia is typified by general difficulty with numbers, recognizing patterns, and sorting objects by shape or size. As children enter school and math learning progresses, the characteristics may include trouble with simple addition, subtraction, multiplication, and division, as well as difficulty retaining numerical concepts and applying math to common situations.

Teens with dyscalculia continue to have problems as math becomes increasingly complex and more is expected of them. Symptoms for this age group, as well as adults, can include:

It is not unusual for dyscalculia to co-occur with other types of learning difficulties, such as attention deficit hyperactivity disorder (ADHD), dyslexia, or dyspraxia (problems with movement), so evaluation will often include testing for these conditions, as well.

- Lack of understanding of time, often late or miscalculating how long tasks will take
- Difficulty applying math principles to everyday life, such as calculating the area of a room or the amount of a tip
- Poor sense of direction, easily gets lost or worries about getting lost
- Trouble judging distances between objects
- May do well in classes that require reading and writing skills, such as English and history, but struggles in those that rely on numbers, like algebra and science
- Trouble with measurements, as in recipes or woodworking, especially when conversions are necessary (e.g., pints to ounces)
- Difficulty understanding information in chart or graph form
- Good recall of spoken or printed words, but has trouble remembering numbers and patterns

Diagnosis of Dyscalculia

Most often, various types of learning disabilities are identified when children are quite young, and this is usually the case with dyscalculia. But, often younger students do so well in other areas, and the level of math being taught is simple enough, that they are able to mask the symptoms. As a result, in some cases dyscalculia may not be diagnosed until the teen years, when work with numbers becomes considerably more complex and students start to fall behind.

There is no single cause for dyscalculia, but because some of the underlying problems can be neurological or genetic, the first step in diagnosis should be a physical examination by a doctor who is aware that the teen has been exhibiting some of the above symptoms. If no physical cause can be determined, then the student should be evaluated by a specialist in learning disabilities, who will review past performance, administer a variety of tests, and ask questions to determine the individual's skills and understanding of various concepts. Some of the evaluation process will likely include:

- Questions about areas in which the teen feels she or he has had difficulty
- Questions about times when the student has felt hopeless or frustrated about math
- Probing for other learning disabilities that may be contributing factors
- An evaluation of basic math skills (counting, addition, subtraction, etc.)

Students who have been diagnosed with dyscalculia may be eligible for special classroom accommodation or other support under the Individuals with Disabilities Education Act (IDEA). Ask a school guidance counselor, special education teacher, or the principal's office for more information.
(Source: "Dyslexia and Specific Learning Disabilities," U.S. Department of Education (ED))

- Determining whether the teen can discern patterns and organize objects logically
- Testing for the ability to estimate quantity
- Gauging the individual's facility with money (making change, estimating costs, etc.)
- Evaluating the ability to tell time and determine how long tasks will take
- Assessing the student's ability to find alternate ways to solve problems

An important part of diagnosis is to evaluate how well the teen is able to understand math concepts and apply them to common situations, rather than just having her or him perform a series of calculations. For math learning to move forward, it is critical that the student develop a solid grasp of underlying principles, and this would not happen without an accurate assessment of her or his history and current status.

Treatment of Dyscalculia

Dyscalculia cannot be cured, and it would not improve on its own. But, with treatment by a trained professional, along with dedication on the part of the student and support from teachers, parents, and peers, math skills can be improved considerably. Some strategies include:

- Helping students be aware of their strengths and weaknesses so they can understand and make use of their own unique learning style
- Devising real-life examples that link math skills to everyday situations
- Breaking complex problems into smaller, more easily managed parts
- Using visual aids, such as drawings or physical objects, to help solve math problems
- Talking through the problem-solving process verbally
- Using graph paper to help organize ideas
- Working on a calculator when this is appropriate
- Circling computation signs before trying to solve a problem
- Covering up most of a math exercise or test with a piece of paper to make it easier to concentrate on one problem at a time
- Playing math-related video games
- Reading math problems aloud and continuing to talk while working on a solution

- Reviewing new skills, discussing, and asking questions before moving on to the next task
- Engaging a tutor to help with review, practice, and any particular areas of difficulty
- Working with a classmate or other peer on homework assignments or to review the day's lessons

References

1. "Dyscalculia," National Center for Learning Disabilities (NCLD), 2007.
2. "Dyscalculia: Indications, Treatment and Strategies," NoBullying.com, September 4, 2016.
3. Morin, Amanda. "Treatment Options for Dyscalculia," Understood.org, n.d.
4. Morin, Amanda. "Understanding Dyscalculia," Understood.org, n.d.
5. "What Is Dyscalculia?" Dyslexia SPELD Foundation, 2014.

CHAPTER 15
READING AND WRITING DISABILITIES

About This Chapter: Text in this chapter begins with excerpts from "About Reading and Reading Disorders," *Eunice Kennedy Shriver* National Institute of Child Health and Human Development (NICHD), March 5, 2020; Text under the heading "About Dysgraphia: Writing Disability" is excerpted from "Dysgraphia Information Page," National Institute of Neurological Disorders and Stroke (NINDS), March 27, 2019.

About Reading Disorders
What Are Reading Disorders?

Reading disorders occur when a person has trouble reading words or understanding what they read. Dyslexia is one type of reading disorder. It generally refers to difficulties reading individual words and can lead to problems understanding text.

Most reading disorders result from specific differences in the way the brain processes written words and text. Usually, these differences are present from a young age. But, a person can develop a reading problem from an injury to the brain at any age.

People with reading disorders often have problems recognizing words they already know and understanding text they read. They also may be poor spellers. Not everyone with a reading disorder has every symptom.

Reading disorders are not a type of intellectual or developmental disorder, and they are not a sign of lower intelligence or unwillingness to learn.

People with reading disorders may have other learning disabilities, too, including problems with writing or numbers.

Types of Reading Disorders

Dyslexia is the most well-known reading disorder. It specifically impairs a person's ability to read. Individuals with dyslexia have normal intelligence, but they read at levels significantly lower than expected. Although the disorder varies from person to person, there are common characteristics: people with dyslexia often have a hard time sounding out words, understanding written words, and naming objects quickly.

Reading is the process by which a person gets information from written symbols like letters, characters, and words. A person can read using sight or touch, such as when a vision-impaired person reads braille.

Most reading problems are present from the time a child learns to read. But, some people lose the ability to read after a stroke or an injury to the area of the brain involved with reading. This kind of reading disorder is called **"alexia."**

Hyperlexia is a disorder where people have advanced reading skills, but may have problems understanding what is read or spoken aloud. They may also have cognitive or social problems.

Other people may have normal reading skills, but have problems understanding written words.

Reading disorders can also involve problems with specific skills:

- **Word decoding.** People who have difficulty sounding out written words struggle to match letters to their proper sounds.
- **Fluency.** People who lack fluency have difficulty reading quickly, accurately, and with proper expression (if reading aloud).
- **Poor reading comprehension.** People with poor reading comprehension have trouble understanding what they read.

About Dysgraphia: Writing Disability
What Is Dysgraphia?

Dysgraphia is a neurological disorder characterized by writing disabilities. Specifically, the disorder causes a person's writing to be distorted or incorrect. In children, the disorder generally emerges when they are first introduced to writing. They make inappropriately sized and spaced letters, or write wrong or misspelled words, despite thorough instruction. Children with the disorder may have other learning disabilities; however, they usually have no social or other academic problems. Cases of dysgraphia in adults generally occur after some trauma. In addition to poor handwriting, dysgraphia is characterized by wrong or odd spelling, and production of words that are not correct (i.e., using "boy" for "child"). The cause of the disorder is unknown, but in adults, it is usually associated with damage to the parietal lobe of the brain.

Treatment of Dysgraphia

Treatment for dysgraphia varies and may include treatment for motor disorders to help control writing movements. Other treatments may address impaired memory or other neurological problems. Some physicians recommend that individuals with dysgraphia use computers to avoid the problems of handwriting.

Prognosis of Dysgraphia

Some individuals with dysgraphia improve their writing ability, but for others, the disorder persists.

CHAPTER 16
SPECIFIC LANGUAGE IMPAIRMENT

About This Chapter: This chapter includes text excerpted from "Specific Language Impairment," National Institute on Deafness and Other Communication Disorders (NIDCD), October 21, 2019.

What Is Specific Language Impairment?

Specific language impairment (SLI) is a communication disorder that interferes with the development of language skills in children who have no hearing loss or intellectual disabilities. SLI can affect a child's speaking, listening, reading, and writing. SLI is also called "developmental language disorder," "language delay," or "developmental dysphasia." It is one of the most common developmental disorders, affecting approximately seven to eight percent of children in kindergarten. The impact of SLI usually persists into adulthood.

What Causes Specific Language Impairment

The cause of SLI is unknown, but discoveries suggest that it has a strong genetic link. Children with SLI are more likely than those without SLI to have parents and siblings who have also had difficulties and delays in speaking. In fact, 50 to 70 percent of children with SLI have at least one family member with the disorder.

Learning more than one language at a time does not cause SLI. The disorder can, however, affect both multilingual children and children who speak only one language.

What Are the Symptoms of Specific Language Impairment?

A child with SLI often has a history of being a late talker (reaching spoken language milestones later than peers).

Preschool-aged children with SLI may:
- Be late to put words together into sentences
- Struggle to learn new words and make conversation

- Have difficulty following directions, not because they are stubborn, but because they do not fully understand the words spoken to them
- Make frequent grammatical errors when speaking

Although some late talkers eventually catch up with peers, children with SLI have persistent language difficulties. Symptoms common in older children and adults with SLI include:
- Limited use of complex sentences
- Difficulty finding the right words
- Difficulty understanding figurative language
- Reading problems
- Disorganized storytelling and writing
- Frequent grammatical and spelling errors

How Is Specific Language Impairment Diagnosed?

If a doctor, teacher, or parent suspects that a child has SLI, a speech-language pathologist (a professional trained to assess and treat people with speech or language problems) can evaluate the child's language skills. The type of evaluation depends on the child's age and the concerns that led to the evaluation. In general, an evaluation includes:
- Direct observation of the child
- Interviews and questionnaires completed by parents and/or teachers
- Assessments of the child's learning ability
- Standardized tests of current language performance

These tools allow the speech-language pathologist to compare the child's language skills to those of same-age peers, identify specific difficulties, and plan for potential treatment targets.

Is Specific Language Impairment the Same Thing as a Learning Disability?

Specific language impairment is not the same thing as a learning disability. Instead, SLI is a risk factor for learning disabilities, since problems with basic language skills affect classroom performance. This means that children with SLI are more likely to be diagnosed with a learning disability than children who do not have SLI. They may struggle with translating letters into sounds for reading. Their writing skills may be weakened by grammatical errors, limited vocabulary, and problems with comprehension and organizing thoughts into coherent sentences. Difficulties with language comprehension can make mathematical word problems challenging. Some children with SLI may show signs of dyslexia. By the time they reach adulthood, people with SLI are six times more likely to be diagnosed with reading and spelling disabilities and four times more likely to be diagnosed with math disabilities than those who do not have SLI.

Is Specific Language Impairment a Lifelong Condition?

Specific language impairment is a developmental disorder, which means that its symptoms first appear in childhood. This does not mean that, as children develop, they grow out of the problem. Instead, the problem is apparent in early childhood and will likely continue, but change, with development.

For instance, a young child with SLI might use ungrammatical sentences in conversation, while a young adult with SLI might avoid complex sentences in conversations and struggle to produce clear, concise, well-organized, and grammatically accurate writing.

Early treatment during the preschool years can improve the skills of many children with language delays, including those with SLI. Children who enter kindergarten with significant language delays are likely to continue having problems, but they and even older children can still benefit from treatment. Many adults develop strategies for managing SLI symptoms. This can improve their daily social, family, and work lives.

What Treatments Are Available for Specific Language Impairment?

Treatment services for SLI are typically provided or overseen by a licensed speech-language pathologist. Treatment may be provided in homes, schools, university programs for speech-language pathology, private clinics, or outpatient hospital settings.

Identifying and treating children with SLI early in life is ideal, but people can respond well to treatment regardless of when it begins. Treatment depends on the age and needs of the person. Starting treatment early can help young children to:

- Acquire missing elements of grammar
- Expand their understanding and use of words
- Develop social communication skills

For school-age children, treatment may focus on understanding instruction in the classroom, including helping with issues such as:

- Following directions
- Understanding the meaning of the words that teachers use
- Organizing information
- Improving speaking, reading, and writing skills

Adults entering new jobs, vocational programs, or higher education may need help learning technical vocabulary or improving workplace writing skills.

CHAPTER 17
NONVERBAL LEARNING DISABILITY

About This Chapter: "Nonverbal Learning Disability," © 2016 Omnigraphics. Reviewed July 2020.

Nonverbal learning disability (NLD) is a brain-based learning disability where individuals have difficulty with abstract thinking, spatial relationships, and identifying and interpreting concepts and patterns. Nonverbal learning disability occurs in 0.1 to 1 percent of the general population. It is also called "nonverbal learning disorder" (NVLD) or a "right-hemisphere learning disorder."

People use the spoken word in various ways. Sometimes they say exactly what they mean. Sometimes they expect the listener to pick up another meaning from their facial expression or tone of voice. Sometimes they expect the listener to fill in information from past experience or some other source of information. For example "I love rainy days" when said directly is the truth. But, if the same phrase is said with a frown or eye roll and a growly tone, the speaker is being sarcastic, and is really telling the listener that she hates rainy days. Finally, if the speaker says, "You know how I feel about rainy days," the listener is expected to fill in some previously learned information. A person with a nonverbal learning disability cannot interpret the facial expressions and tone of voice of the sarcasm and thus takes the untrue statement as true. Nor can the listener draw on a pattern of previously learned information, and thus truly does not know how the speaker feels.

Signs of Nonverbal Learning Disability

Children with NLD tend to be very smart. They talk freely, develop large vocabularies in comparison to other children of their age, memorize facts, and read early. Intelligence tests show high verbal intelligence quotient (IQ) but low-performance IQ due to visual-spatial difficulties.

There are five main areas of weakness in people with NLD. People with NLD may not exhibit weakness in all five areas, nor may they exhibit them all at once. The weaknesses tend to become more obvious as children progress in school and are required to rely more on identifying patterns and less on memorized facts.

The five main areas of weakness have been identified as:

- **Visual/spatial awareness.** Children with NLD may have problems estimating distance, size, and/or shape of objects. They may be clumsy, spill drinks, bump into people or objects, or not be able to catch a ball. They may also have a poor sense of direction, such as being able to distinguish left from right.
- **Motor skills.** Children with NLD may have trouble mastering basic motor skills both large (such as dressing themselves, running, or riding a bike) or small (such as writing or using scissors).
- **Abstract thinking.** Children with NLD may have difficulty seeing or understanding the big picture. They can read a story and relate the details, but cannot answer questions about how the details fit together.
- **Conceptual skills.** Children with NLD may have trouble grasping the larger concept of a situation. For example, determining how pieces of a puzzle fit together to make a whole or identifying the steps needed to solve a problem. This contributes to problems especially with math.
- **Social skills.** Children with NLD may have trouble making friends or socializing in a group. They may interrupt or behave inappropriately in social situations. They use previously learned skills to cope with new social situations, whether appropriate or not.

In addition, because NLD occurs in the right side of the brain, children with NLD may have a distorted sense of touch or feel and poor coordination on the left side of the body.

These areas of weakness are often masked in preschool and the early elementary grades when students are learning basic (rote) skills like reading and arithmetic. By the fourth or fifth grade, when students are required to process what they read or remember patterns from previous examples, the weaknesses start to become evident. At the same time, these very smart children may start exhibiting behavioral problems brought on by frustration in not "getting it" or feelings of being a social reject.

Diagnosis of Nonverbal Learning Disability

The diagnosis of NLD is controversial. NLD is not listed in the American Psychiatric Association's (APA) *Diagnostic and Statistical Manual of Mental Disorders, 5th ed.*, the manual used by doctors and therapists to diagnose learning disabilities. Nor is NLD recognized as a disability covered by the Individuals with Disabilities Education Act (IDEA). Nonetheless, if a child is exhibiting signs of NLD, there are steps parents should take to identify the problem.

- **A medical exam.** A thorough physical examination and a discussion of the child's learning problems will help the doctor rule out any physical causes for the learning problems.

- **A mental-health professional.** Most likely the family doctor will refer the child to a neurologist or other specialist. The specialist will talk to the parents and child about what is happening, and may administer a variety of tests in the areas of speech and language, motor skills, and visual-spatial relationships. The results coupled with information from the parents and child will help the specialist analyze the strengths and weaknesses associated with NLD and make a diagnosis.

As with many learning disorders, the symptoms of NLD vary from child to child, thus a comprehensive assessment is needed to determine the individual child's needs. With the input and support of learning professionals and therapists as well as the family, steps can be taken to help the student with NLD.

Help for Those with Nonverbal Learning Disability

It is important to work with the child's school specialists to develop accommodations for the child's NLD. Formal accommodations may be developed through an Individualized Education Program (IEP) or 504 plan. If the child does not qualify for either plan, informal accommodations may be made in the classroom. Classroom accommodations may include modifying homework assignments, tests for time and content, and presenting lectures with PowerPoint slides so the student can see as well as hear the material being covered, and/or working with a reading specialist to read a passage aloud then extract key terms and ideas.

Parents can help their child in various ways that will make things easier for both the student and the family. They can:
- Establish structure and routine
- Give clear instructions
- Keep a chart of the day's activities, both social and academic
- Make transitions easier by giving logical, step-by-step explanations of what is going to happen (We are going to IHOP for dinner. We need to leave in an hour.)
- Break down tasks into small steps in a logical sequence
- Play games with the child to have her or him identify emotions from facial expressions or voice tone
- Avoid sarcasm, or if it happens, use the experience to help the child identify the signs of sarcasm
- Set up one-on-one play dates with another child who shares an interest with yours. Play dates should be structured, monitored, and time bound.
- Avoid situations that may overwhelm the child with too much sensory input—noise, smell, activity

There are other sources of help for parents and students. Social skills groups help the student in social situations. Parent behavioral training helps parents learn how to collaborate with teachers. Occupational and physical therapy may help the child improve movement and writing skills as well as build tolerance for outside experiences. Cognitive therapy can help the child deal with anxiety, depression, and other mental-health issues.

Although NLD presents many challenges for both the student and the family, there is help available and with patience and effort, there will be improvement.

References

1. Epstein, Varda. "Nonverbal Learning Disorder: Is This What Your Child Has?" Kars4Kids, July 1, 2015.
2. Miller, Caroline. "What Is Nonverbal Learning Disorder?" Child Mind Institute, 2016.
3. Patino, Erica. "Understanding Nonverbal Learning Disabilities," Understood. org, May 21, 2014.
4. "Quick Facts on Nonverbal Learning Disorder," Child Mind Institute, 2016.
5. Thompson, Sue. "Nonverbal Learning Disorders," LD online, 1996.

CHAPTER 18
DEVELOPMENTAL GERSTMANN SYNDROME

About This Chapter: This chapter includes text excerpted from "Gerstmann Syndrome Information Page," National Institute of Neurological Disorders and Stroke (NINDS), March 27, 2019.

What Is Gerstmann Syndrome?

Gerstmann syndrome is a cognitive impairment that results from damage to a specific area of the brain—the left parietal lobe in the region of the angular gyrus. It may occur after a stroke or in association with damage to the parietal lobe. It is characterized by four primary symptoms: a writing disability (agraphia or dysgraphia), a lack of understanding of the rules for calculation or arithmetic (acalculia or dyscalculia), an inability to distinguish right from left, and an inability to identify fingers (finger agnosia). The disorder should not be confused with Gerstmann-Sträussler-Scheinker (GSS) disease, a type of transmissible spongiform encephalopathy.

In addition to exhibiting the above symptoms, many adults also experience aphasia, (difficulty in expressing oneself when speaking, in understanding speech, or in reading and writing).

There are few reports of the syndrome, sometimes called "developmental Gerstmann syndrome," in children. The cause is not known. Most cases are identified when children reach school age, a time when they are challenged with writing and math exercises. Generally, children with the disorder exhibit poor handwriting and spelling skills, and difficulty with math functions, including adding, subtracting, multiplying, and dividing. An inability to differentiate right from left and to discriminate among individual fingers may also be apparent. In addition to the four primary symptoms, many children also suffer from constructional apraxia, an inability to copy simple drawings. Frequently, there is also an impairment in reading. Children with a high level of intellectual functioning as well as those with brain damage may be affected with the disorder.

Treatment of Gerstmann Syndrome

There is no cure for Gerstmann syndrome. Treatment is symptomatic and supportive. Occupational and speech therapies may help diminish the dysgraphia and apraxia. In addition, calculators and word processors may help school children cope with the symptoms of the disorder.

Prognosis of Gerstmann Syndrome

In adults, many of the symptoms diminish over time. Although it has been suggested that in children symptoms may diminish over time, it appears likely that most children probably do not overcome their deficits, but learn to adjust to them.

CHAPTER 19

DEVELOPMENTAL DYSPRAXIA: IMPAIRED SENSORY AND MOTOR SKILLS

About This Chapter: This chapter includes text excerpted from "Developmental Dyspraxia Information Page," National Institute of Neurological Disorders and Stroke (NINDS), March 27, 2019.

What Is Developmental Dyspraxia?

Developmental dyspraxia is a disorder characterized by an impairment in the ability to plan and carry out sensory and motor tasks. Generally, individuals with the disorder appear "out of sync" with their environment. Symptoms vary and may include poor balance and coordination, clumsiness, vision problems, perception difficulties, emotional and behavioral problems, difficulty with reading, writing, and speaking, poor social skills, poor posture, and poor short-term memory. Although individuals with the disorder may be of average or above-average intelligence, they may behave immaturely.

Treatment of Developmental Dyspraxia

Treatment is symptomatic and supportive and may include occupational and speech therapy, and "cueing" or other forms of communication such as using pictures and hand gestures. Many children with the disorder require special education.

Prognosis of Developmental Dyspraxia

Developmental dyspraxia is a lifelong disorder. Many individuals are able to compensate for their disabilities through occupational and speech therapy.

CHAPTER 20
DISRUPTION IN EXECUTIVE FUNCTION

About This Chapter: This chapter includes text excerpted from "Executive Function," Administration for Children and Families (ACF), U.S. Department of Health and Human Services (HHS), January 11, 2017.

What Is Executive Function?

Executive functions or self-regulation serves as the foundation for life-long functioning in areas such as critical thinking and problem-solving, planning, decision making, and executing tasks. Executive functions or self-regulatory capacities are the building blocks for a range of important skills. These skills mature at different rates and develop over time. Working memory and self-control are among the first set of executive functions that develop (typically during the early childhood), setting the stage for attentional capacities and goal-directed behavior during the preteens years, better planning and refined goal-directed behavior during adolescence, and more efficient problem-solving, decision making, and cognitive flexibility in adulthood.

The experience of trauma, especially when it is prolonged, can disrupt executive functioning skills. Children who have experienced prolonged or pronounced stress and adversity, including poverty and trauma experiences, may struggle more than other children do to regulate their thoughts, feelings, and behaviors. Severe childhood stress appears to have lasting effects, with executive function or self-regulation related difficulties seen into adulthood. In addition, adolescents who report having experienced trauma, such as maltreatment or exposure to a parent's intimate partner violence, have been found to be less effective than their peers at controlling their attention, regulating their emotions, and planning. Adults whose overall functioning has been compromised by adversity and continued stress are less likely to engage in intentional self-regulation, and have difficulty with problem-solving, and impulse control. Less is known about the effects of trauma in adulthood on executive functioning and related skills.

Why the Concept of Executive Function is Important to Human Services

Executive functions involve regions of the brain associated with information processing, (including such functions as attention and working memory), regulating emotions and behavior (including such functions as impulse control and suppressing inappropriate responses), and even creativity and some aspects of personality. Individuals who have problems with executive functions in childhood or adulthood may have difficulty with social appropriateness, planning projects, working independently, remembering details, paying attention, or starting and completing tasks.

Human service agencies can strive to build and enhance executive functioning skills for the children, youth and adults served in their programs. For individuals who are also impacted by toxic stress, trauma and other adverse experiences, improved executive functioning skills will be needed to promote engagement and participation in human service programs. Children and adults who can develop these skills may be better able to benefit from programs and services provided by human services agencies.

Developmental perspective. It is important for human service agencies to keep in mind that executive functioning skills change across development from infancy through late life. For example, programs serving infants from birth to three years may be designed to support the child's ability to maintain focus and attention, show persistence in actions, and demonstrate an ability to be flexible in actions and behavior. Preschool programs may target increasing the child's ability to control impulses, maintaining focus, persisting in tasks, holding information, and demonstrating flexibility in thinking and behavior. Programs serving older children may target additional developmentally appropriate skills and abilities, including planning, problem-solving, and organizing. In adolescence and adulthood, programs may address reasoning, goal setting, and decision-making. Agencies focused on supportive care for older adults may offer cognitive health promotion programs that enhance cognition, memory, and inhibitory control.

Relevant Interventions and Approaches

A wide range of activities requires executive functioning skills, and targeted interventions may foster these skills. Interventions to improve executive functions include programs to train working memory, mindfulness programs to help address focus and attention, providing routine structure and organization to facilitate task completion as well coaching to motivate behavior. However, it is important to consider carefully how executive functioning and other regulation-related skills are defined and measured in research and evaluation. Programs that improve one specific skill will not necessarily lead to improvements in other related skills.

Human services agencies offer a range of social services and support for individuals, children and families, and adults throughout the lifespan. While the programs may differ in terms of target population, services provided, and outcomes expected, a general understanding of how executive functioning and self-regulation skills can foster optimal health, development and well-being, will be important for all programs and staff. Human services agencies are well-positioned to use information about the importance of executive functioning skills in program planning, design, implementation, staff development, and family engagement efforts.

PART 3 | CONGENITAL AND GENETIC DISORDERS THAT AFFECT LEARNING

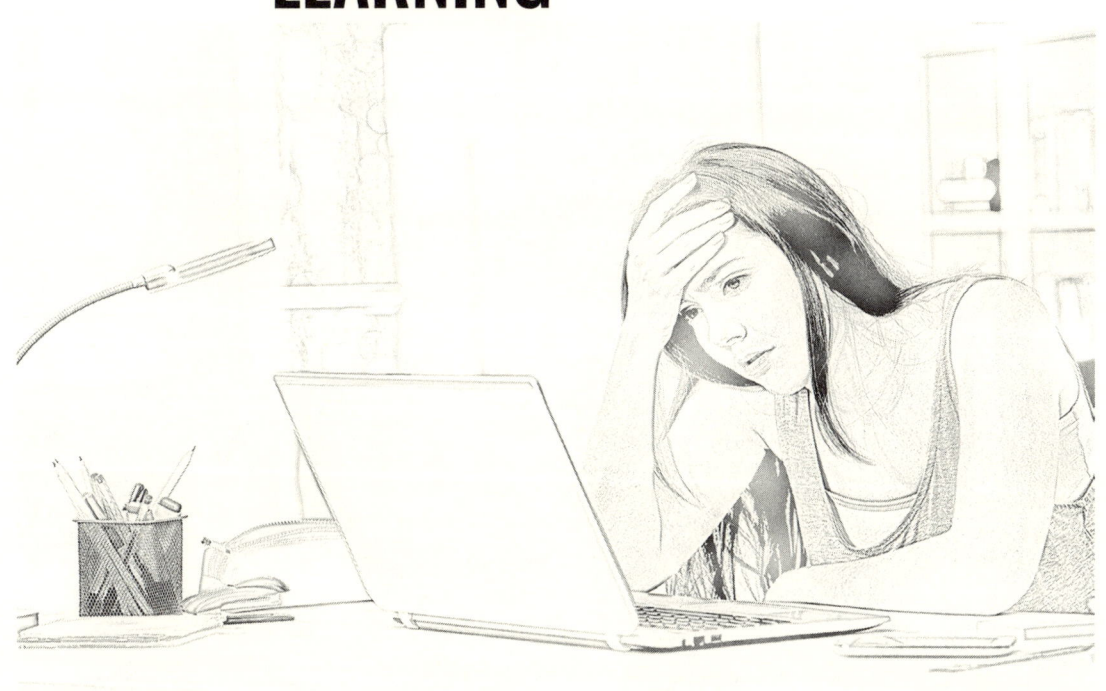

CHAPTER 21
FETAL ALCOHOL SPECTRUM DISORDERS

About This Chapter: This chapter includes text excerpted from "Basics about FASDs," Centers for Disease Control and Prevention (CDC), May 7, 2020.

Fetal alcohol spectrum disorders (FASDs) are a group of conditions that can occur in a person whose mother drank alcohol during pregnancy. These effects can include physical problems and problems with behavior and learning. Often, a person with an FASD has a mix of these problems.

Cause and Prevention of Fetal Alcohol Spectrum Disorders

Fetal alcohol spectrum disorders are caused by a woman drinking alcohol during pregnancy. Alcohol in the mother's blood passes to the baby through the umbilical cord.

There is no known safe amount of alcohol during pregnancy or when trying to get pregnant. There is also no safe time to drink during pregnancy. Alcohol can cause problems for a developing baby throughout pregnancy, including before a woman knows she is pregnant. All types of alcohol are equally harmful, including all wines and beer.

To prevent a child from having an FASD, a woman should not drink alcohol while she is pregnant, or might be pregnant. This is because a woman could get pregnant and not know for up to four to six weeks.

If a woman is drinking alcohol during pregnancy, it is never too late to stop drinking. Because brain growth takes place throughout pregnancy, the sooner a woman stops drinking the better it will be for her and her baby.

Fetal alcohol spectrum disorders are preventable if a woman does not drink alcohol during pregnancy.

Signs and Symptoms of Fetal Alcohol Spectrum Disorders

Fetal alcohol spectrum disorders refer to a collection of diagnoses that represent the range of effects that can happen to a person whose mother drank alcohol during pregnancy. These conditions can affect each person in different ways, and can range from mild-to-severe.

A person with an FASD might have:

- Low body weight
- Poor coordination
- Hyperactive behavior
- Difficulty with attention
- Poor memory
- Difficulty in school (especially with math)
- Learning disabilities
- Speech and language delays
- Intellectual disability or low IQ
- Poor reasoning and judgment skills
- Sleep and sucking problems as a baby
- Vision or hearing problems
- Problems with the heart, kidneys, or bones
- Shorter-than-average height
- Small head size
- Abnormal facial features, such as a smooth ridge between the nose and upper lip (this ridge is called the "philtrum")

Diagnosis of Fetal Alcohol Spectrum Disorders

Different FASD diagnoses are based on particular symptoms and include:

- **Fetal alcohol syndrome (FAS).** FAS represents the most involved end of the FASD spectrum. People with FAS have central nervous system (CNS) problems, minor facial features, and growth problems. People with FAS can have problems with learning, memory, attention span, communication, vision, or hearing. They might have a mix of these problems. People with FAS often have a hard time in school and trouble getting along with others.
- **Alcohol-related neurodevelopmental disorder (ARND).** People with ARND might have intellectual disabilities and problems with behavior and learning. They might do poorly in school and have difficulties with math, memory, attention, judgment, and poor impulse control.
- **Alcohol-related birth defects (ARBD).** People with ARBD might have problems with the heart, kidneys, or bones or with hearing. They might have a mix of these.
  - **Neurobehavioral disorder associated with prenatal alcohol exposure (ND-PAE).** ND-PAE was first included as a recognized condition in the *Diagnostic and Statistical Manual of Mental Disorders, Fifth Edition* (*DSM 5*) of the American Psychiatric Association (APA) in 2013. A child or youth with ND-PAE will have problems in three areas:
    - Thinking and memory, where the child may have trouble planning or may forget material she or he has already learned

The term "fetal alcohol effects" (FAE) was previously used to describe intellectual disabilities and problems with behavior and learning in a person whose mother drank alcohol during pregnancy. In 1996, the Institute of Medicine (IOM) replaced FAE with the terms ARND and ARBD.

- Behavior problems, such as severe tantrums, mood issues (e.g., irritability), and difficulty shifting attention from one task to another
- Trouble with day-to-day living, which can include problems with bathing, dressing for the weather, and playing with other children. In addition, to be diagnosed with ND-PAE, the mother of the child must have consumed more than minimal levels of alcohol before the child's birth, which APA defines as more than 13 alcoholic drinks per month of pregnancy (i.e., any 30-day period of pregnancy) or more than two alcoholic drinks in one sitting.

Areas Evaluated for Fetal Alcohol Spectrum Disorders Diagnoses

The term FASDs is not meant for use as a clinical diagnosis.

Diagnosing FASDs can be hard because there is no medical test, such as a blood test, for these conditions. And other disorders, such as attention deficit hyperactivity disorder (ADHD) and Williams syndrome, have some symptoms like fetal alcohol syndrome (FAS).

To diagnose FASDs, doctors look for:
- Prenatal alcohol exposure; although confirmation is not required to make a diagnosis
- Central nervous system problems (e.g., small head size, problems with attention and hyperactivity, poor coordination)
- Lower-than-average height, weight, or both
- Abnormal facial features (e.g., smooth ridge between nose and upper lip)

Treatment of Fetal Alcohol Spectrum Disorders

Fetal alcohol spectrum disorders last a lifetime. There is no cure for FASDs, but research shows that early intervention treatment services can improve a child's development.

There are many types of treatment options, including medication to help with some symptoms, behavior and education therapy, parent training, and other alternative approaches. No one treatment is right for every child. Good treatment plans will include close monitoring, follow-ups, and changes as needed along the way.

Also, "protective factors" can help reduce the effects of FASDs and help people with these conditions reach their full potential.

Protective factors include:
- Diagnosis before six years of age
- Loving, nurturing, and stable home environment during the school years
- Absence of violence
- Involvement in special education and social services

Get Help!

If you or the doctor thinks there could be a problem, **ask the doctor for a referral to a specialist** (someone who knows about FASDs), such as a developmental pediatrician, child psychologist, or clinical geneticist. In some cities, there are clinics whose staff have special training in diagnosing and treating children with FASDs. To find doctors and clinics in your area visit the National and State Resource Directory (www.nofas.org/resource-directory) from the National Organization on Fetal Alcohol Syndrome (NOFAS).

At the same time as you ask the doctor for a referral to a specialist, **call your state or territory's early intervention program** to request a free evaluation to find out if your child can get services to help. This is sometimes called a "*Child Find*" evaluation. You do not need to wait for a doctor's referral or a medical diagnosis to make this call.

Where to call for a free evaluation from the state depends on your child's age:

- **If your child is younger than three years old.** Call your state or territory's early intervention program (www.cdc.gov/ncbddd/actearly/parents/states.html) and say: "I have concerns about my child's development and I would like to have my child evaluated to find out if she/he is eligible for early intervention services."
- **If your child is three years old or older.** Contact your local public school system. Even if your child is not old enough for kindergarten or enrolled in a public school, call your local elementary school or board of education and ask to speak with someone who can help you have your child evaluated.

CHAPTER 22
DOWN SYNDROME AND LEARNING DIFFICULTIES

About This Chapter: Text beginning with the heading "What Is Down Syndrome?" is excerpted from "Facts about Down Syndrome," Centers for Disease Control and Prevention (CDC), December 5, 2019; Text beginning with the heading "Is There a Cure for Down Syndrome?" is excerpted from "Down Syndrome: Other FAQs," *Eunice Kennedy Shriver* National Institute of Child Health and Human Development (NICHD), January 31, 2017.

What Is Down Syndrome?

Down syndrome (DS) is a condition in which a person has an extra chromosome. Chromosomes are small "packages" of genes in the body. They determine how a baby's body forms during pregnancy and how the baby's body functions as it grows in the womb and after birth. Typically, a baby is born with 46 chromosomes. Babies with DS have an extra copy of one of these chromosomes, chromosome 21. A medical term for having an extra copy of a chromosome is 'trisomy.' DS is also referred to as "Trisomy 21." This extra copy changes how the baby's body and brain develop, which can cause both mental and physical challenges for the baby.

Even though people with DS might act and look similar, each person has different abilities. People with DS usually have an IQ (a measure of intelligence) in the mildly-to-moderately low range and are slower to speak than other children.

Some common physical features of DS include:

- A flattened face, especially the bridge of the nose
- Almond-shaped eyes that slant up
- A short neck
- Small ears
- A tongue that tends to stick out of the mouth
- Tiny white spots on the iris (colored part) of the eye
- Small hands and feet
- A single line across the palm of the hand (palmar crease)

89

- Small pinky fingers that sometimes curve toward the thumb
- Poor muscle tone or loose joints
- Shorter in height as children and adults

How Many Babies Are Born with Down Syndrome?

Down syndrome remains the most common chromosomal condition diagnosed in the United States. Each year, about 6,000 babies born in the United States have DS. This means that DS occurs in about 1 in every 700 babies.

Types of Down Syndrome

There are three types of DS. People often cannot tell the difference between each type without looking at the chromosomes because the physical features and behaviors are similar.

- **Trisomy 21.** About 95 percent of people with DS have Trisomy 21. With this type of DS, each cell in the body has three separate copies of chromosome 21 instead of the usual two copies.
- **Translocation Down syndrome.** This type accounts for a small percentage of people with DS (about 3%). This occurs when an extra part or a whole extra chromosome 21 is present, but it is attached or "trans-located" to a different chromosome rather than being a separate chromosome 21.
- **Mosaic Down syndrome.** This type affects about two percent of the people with DS. Mosaic means mixture or combination. For children with mosaic DS, some of their cells have three copies of chromosome 21, but other cells have the typical two copies of chromosome 21. Children with mosaic DS may have the same features as other children with DS. However, they may have fewer features of the condition due to the presence of some (or many) cells with a typical number of chromosomes.

Causes and Risk Factors of Down Syndrome

- The extra chromosome 21 leads to the physical features and developmental challenges that can occur among people with DS. Researchers know that DS is caused by an extra chromosome, but no one knows for sure why DS occurs or how many different factors play a role.
- One factor that increases the risk for having a baby with DS is the mother's age. Women who are 35 years or older when they become pregnant are more likely to have a pregnancy affected by DS than women who become pregnant at a younger age. However, the majority of babies with DS are born to mothers less than 35 years old, because there are many more births among younger women.

Diagnosis of Down Syndrome

There are two basic types of tests available to detect DS during pregnancy: screening tests and diagnostic tests. A screening test can tell a woman and her healthcare

In recent years, noninvasive prenatal testing (NIPT) has become available to women who are at increased risk to have a baby with DS. NIPT is a blood test that examines deoxyribonucleic acid (DNA) from the fetus in the mother's bloodstream. However, women who have a positive NIPT result should then have invasive diagnostic testing to confirm the result.

(Source: "Down Syndrome," Genetic and Rare Diseases Information Center (GARD), National Center for Advancing Translational Sciences (NCATS))

provider whether her pregnancy has a lower or higher chance of having DS. Screening tests do not provide an absolute diagnosis, but they are safer for the mother and the developing baby. Diagnostic tests can typically detect whether or not a baby will have DS, but they can be more risky for the mother and developing baby. Neither screening or diagnostic tests can predict the full impact of DS on a baby; no one can predict this.

Screening Tests

Screening tests often include a combination of a blood test, which measures the amount of various substances in the mother's blood (e.g., MS-AFP, Triple Screen, Quad-screen), and an ultrasound, which creates a picture of the baby. During an ultrasound, one of the things the technician looks at is the fluid behind the baby's neck. Extra fluid in this region could indicate a genetic problem. These screening tests can help determine the baby's risk of DS. Rarely, screening tests can give an abnormal result even when there is nothing wrong with the baby. Sometimes, the test results are normal and yet they miss a problem that does exist.

Diagnostic Tests

Diagnostic tests are usually performed after a positive screening test in order to confirm a DS diagnosis. Types of diagnostic tests include:

- Chorionic villus sampling (CVS)—examines material from the placenta
- Amniocentesis—examines the amniotic fluid (the fluid from the sac surrounding the baby)
- Percutaneous umbilical blood sampling (PUBS)—examines blood from the umbilical cord

These tests look for changes in the chromosomes that would indicate a DS diagnosis.

Other Health Problems

Many people with DS have the common facial features and no other major birth defects. However, some people with DS might have one or more major birth defects or other medical problems. Some of the more common health problems among children with DS are listed below.

Early intervention services, quality educational programs, a stimulating home environment, good healthcare, and positive support from family and friends can help people with DS develop to their full potential. The overall goal of treatment is to boost cognition by improving learning, memory, and speech. Other treatments depend on the specific health problems or complications present in each affected person.

(Source: "Down Syndrome," Genetic and Rare Diseases Information Center (GARD), National Center for Advancing Translational Sciences (NCATS))

- Hearing loss
- Obstructive sleep apnea, which is a condition where the person's breathing temporarily stops while asleep
- Ear infections
- Eye diseases
- Heart defects present at birth

Healthcare providers routinely monitor children with DS for these conditions.

Treatments of Down Syndrome

Down syndrome is a lifelong condition. Services early in life will often help babies and children with DS to improve their physical and intellectual abilities. Most of these services focus on helping children with DS develop to their full potential. These services include speech, occupational, and physical therapy, and they are typically offered through early intervention programs in each state. Children with DS may also need extra help or attention in school, although many children are included in regular classes.

Is There a Cure for Down Syndrome?

Currently, there is no cure for DS. However, researchers are exploring a number of ways to address and correct many aspects of the syndrome.

For example, the *Eunice Kennedy Shriver* National Institute of Child Health and Human Development (NICHD) researchers have used mouse models to test treatments for preventing the intellectual and developmental disabilities associated with DS. One study found that mice with DS who were treated in the womb with specific chemicals had no delay in achieving several developmental milestones. Another study found that specific chemicals prevented learning deficits in adult mice who had DS.

How Can Parents and Providers Help Teens and Young Adults with Down Syndrome Transition into Adulthood?

More and more youth and young adults with DS are achieving some of the same milestones as other young people, such as driving a car and finishing high school. As they start to live more independently, young people with DS get jobs, move into group homes or individual housing, or pursue further education, often at community colleges. Families may need to be advocates to ensure that their young adult children do not "fall through the cracks." Sometimes, young people with DS in the midst of these transitions start to do worse in school or undergo major mood changes. In these cases, additional school assistance or evaluation for hypothyroidism or depression may be appropriate.

Many adolescents and adults with DS find success in jobs. The Americans with Disabilities Act (ADA) makes it illegal for an employer of more than 15 individuals to discriminate against people with disabilities who are qualified to carry out a particular job, and the law requires employers to provide reasonable accommodation. When considering whether their older child with DS might be ready to look for work, parents should keep several factors in mind: Success depends on a healthy sense of self-esteem, the ability to complete tasks without help, a willingness to separate emotionally from family, and access to personal recreational activities. Assistive electronic devices can help, too.

Adolescents often switch from care by a pediatrician to adult care, and this change can be difficult for young people with DS. Families and young people with DS often have strong bonds of trust with their pediatricians, and adult healthcare providers may be poorly prepared to meet the needs of maturing patients with DS. Individuals who receive care at special DS clinics that provide lifelong care might prefer to stay with the providers at these clinics as adults.

Teenagers with DS undergo hormonal changes like any other teen. Parents should encourage their teenagers with DS to develop independent skills in hygiene and self-care, to be aware of privacy issues, and to manage their behavior appropriately. Teenagers with DS also should be educated about puberty, sexuality, sexual activity, and the consequences of such activity. Males with DS generally have a reduced sperm count and are usually unable to father children. In contrast, females with DS have regular menstrual periods and can get pregnant and carry a baby to term. Therefore, healthcare providers and families should consider having discussions with their teens with DS about birth control and preventing sexually transmitted diseases (STDs).

CHAPTER 23

COGNITIVE FEATURES OF KLINEFELTER SYNDROME

About This Chapter: This chapter includes text excerpted from "Klinefelter Syndrome (KS): Condition Information," *Eunice Kennedy Shriver* National Institute of Child Health and Human Development (NICHD), December 1, 2016. Reviewed July 2020.

What Is Klinefelter Syndrome?

The term "Klinefelter syndrome," or "KS," describes a set of features that can occur in a male who is born with an extra X chromosome in his cells. It is named after Dr. Henry Klinefelter, who identified the condition in the 1940s.

Usually, every cell in a male's body, except sperm and red blood cells, contains 46 chromosomes. The 45th and 46th chromosomes—the X and Y chromosomes—are sometimes called "sex chromosomes" because they determine a person's sex. Normally, males have one X and one Y chromosome, making them XY. Males with KS have an extra X chromosome, making them XXY.

Klinefelter syndrome is sometimes called "47,XXY" (47 refers to total chromosomes) or the "XXY condition." Those with KS are sometimes called "XXY males."

Some males with KS may have both XY cells and XXY cells in their bodies. This is called "mosaic." Mosaic males may have fewer symptoms of KS depending on the number of XY cells they have in their bodies and where these cells are located. For example, males who have normal XY cells in their testes may be fertile.

In very rare cases, males might have two or more extra X chromosomes in their cells, for instance XXXY or XXXXY, or an extra Y, such as XXYY. This is called "poly-X Klinefelter syndrome," and it causes more severe symptoms.

What Causes Klinefelter Syndrome

The extra chromosome results from a random error that occurs when a sperm or egg is formed; this error causes an extra X cell to be included each time the cell divides to form new cells. In very rare cases, more than one extra X or an extra Y is included.

Table 23.1. Prevalence of Klinefelter Syndrome Variants

Number of Extra X Chromosomes	One (XXY)	Two (XXXY)	Three (XXXXY)
Number of newborn males with the condition	1 in 500	1 in 50,000	1 in 85,000 to 100,000

How Many People Are Affected By or at Risk for Klinefelter Syndrome?

Researchers estimate that one male in about 500 newborn males has an extra X chromosome, making KS among the most common chromosomal disorders seen in all newborns. The likelihood of a third or fourth X is much rarer:

Scientists are not sure what factors increase the risk of KS. The error that produces the extra chromosome occurs at random, meaning the error is not hereditary or passed down from parent to child. Research suggests that older mothers might be slightly more likely to have a son with KS. However, the extra X chromosome in KS comes from the father about one-half of the time.

What Are Common Symptoms of Klinefelter Syndrome?

Because XXY males do not really appear different from other males and because they may not have any or have mild symptoms, XXY males often do not know they have KS.

In other cases, males with KS may have mild or severe symptoms. Whether or not a male with KS has visible symptoms depends on many factors, including how much testosterone his body makes, if he is mosaic (with both XY and XXY cells), and his age when the condition is diagnosed and treated.

KS symptoms fall into these main categories:

- Physical symptoms
- Language and learning symptoms
- Social and behavioral symptoms
- Symptoms of poly-X KS

Physical Symptoms

Many physical symptoms of KS result from low testosterone levels in the body. The degree of symptoms differs based on the amount of testosterone needed for a specific age or developmental stage and the amount of testosterone the body makes or has available.

During the first few years of life, when the need for testosterone is low, most XXY males do not show any obvious differences from typical male infants and young boys. Some may have slightly weaker muscles, meaning they might sit up, crawl, and walk slightly later than average. For example, on average, baby boys with KS do not start walking until age 18 months.

After age 5 years, when compared to typically developing boys, boys with KS may be slightly:

- Taller
- Fatter around the belly
- Clumsier
- Slower in developing motor skills, coordination, speed, and muscle strength

Puberty for boys with KS usually starts normally. But because their bodies make less testosterone than non-KS boys, their pubertal development may be disrupted or slow. In addition to being tall, KS boys may have:

- Smaller testes and penis
- Breast growth (about one-third of teens with KS have breast growth)
- Less facial and body hair
- Reduced muscle tone
- Narrower shoulders and wider hips
- Weaker bones, greater risk for bone fractures
- Decreased sexual interest
- Lower energy
- Reduced sperm production

An adult male with KS may have these features:

- Infertility: Nearly all men with KS are unable to father a biologically-related child without help from a fertility specialist.
- Small testes, with the possibility of testes shrinking slightly after the teen years
- Lower testosterone levels, which lead to less muscle, hair, and sexual interest and function
- Breasts or breast growth (called "gynecomastia")

In some cases, breast growth can be permanent, and about 10 percent of XXY males need breast-reduction surgery.

Language and Learning Symptoms

Most males with KS have normal intelligence quotients (IQs) and successfully complete education at all levels. (IQ is a frequently used intelligence measure, but does not include emotional, creative, or other types of intelligence.) Between 25 percent and 85 percent of all males with KS have some kind of learning or language-related problem, which makes it more likely that they will need some extra help in school. Without this help or intervention, KS males might fall behind their classmates as schoolwork becomes harder.

KS males may experience some of the following learning and language-related challenges:

- **A delay in learning to talk.** Infants with KS tend to make only a few different vocal sounds. As they grow older, they may have difficulty saying words clearly. It might be hard for them to distinguish differences between similar sounds.
- **Trouble using language to express their thoughts and needs.** Boys with KS might have problems putting their thoughts, ideas, and emotions into words. Some may find it hard to learn and remember some words, such as the names of common objects.
- **Trouble processing what they hear.** Although most boys with KS can understand what is being said to them, they might take longer to process multiple or complex sentences. In some cases, they might fidget or "tune out" because they take longer to process the information. It might also be difficult for KS males to concentrate in noisy settings. They might also be less able to understand a speaker's feelings from just speech alone.
- **Reading difficulties.** Many boys with KS have difficulty understanding what they read (called "poor reading comprehension"). They might also read more slowly than other boys.

By adulthood, most males with KS learn to speak and converse normally, although they may have a harder time doing work that involves extensive reading and writing.

Social and Behavioral Symptoms

Many of the social and behavioral symptoms in KS may result from the language and learning difficulties. For instance, boys with KS who have language difficulties might hold back socially and could use help building social relationships.

Boys with KS, compared to typically developing boys, tend to be:

- Quieter
- Less assertive or self-confident
- More anxious or restless
- Less physically active
- More helpful and eager to please
- More obedient or more ready to follow directions

Symptoms of Poly-X KS

Males with poly-X KS have more than one extra X chromosome, so their symptoms might be more pronounced than in males with KS. In childhood, they may also have seizures, crossed eyes, constipation, and recurrent ear infections. Poly-KS males might also show slight differences in other physical features.

In the teenage years, boys with KS may feel their differences more strongly. As a result, these teen boys are at higher risk of depression, substance abuse, and behavioral disorders. Some teens might withdraw, feel sad, or act out their frustration and anger.

As adults, most men with KS have lives similar to those of men without KS. They successfully complete high school, college, and other levels of education. They have successful and meaningful careers and professions. They have friends and families.

Contrary to research findings published several decades ago, males with KS are no more likely to have serious psychiatric disorders or to get into trouble with the law.

Some common additional symptoms for several poly-X Klinefelter syndromes are listed below.

48,XXYY

- Long legs
- Little body hair
- Lower IQ, average of 60 to 80 (normal IQ is 90 to 110)
- Leg ulcers and other vascular disease symptoms
- Extreme shyness, but also sometimes aggression and impulsiveness

48,XXXY (or Tetrasomy)

- Eyes set further apart
- Flat nose bridge
- Arm bones connected to each other in an unusual way
- Short
- Fifth (smallest) fingers curve inward (clinodactyly)
- Lower IQ, average 40 to 60
- Immature behavior

49,XXXXY (or Pentasomy)

- Low IQ, usually between 20 and 60
- Small head
- Short
- Upward-slanted eyes
- Heart defects, such as when the chambers do not form properly
- High feet arches
- Shy, but friendly
- Difficulty with changing routines

What Are the Treatments for Symptoms in Klinefelter Syndrome?

It is important to remember that because symptoms can be mild, many males with KS are never diagnosed or treated.

The earlier in life that KS symptoms are recognized and treated, the more likely it is that the symptoms can be reduced or eliminated. It is especially helpful to begin treatment by early puberty. Puberty is a time of rapid physical and psychological change, and treatment can successfully limit symptoms. However, treatment can bring benefits at any age.

The type of treatment needed depends on the type of symptoms being treated.
- Treating physical symptoms
- Treating language and learning symptoms
- Treating social and behavioral symptoms

Treating Physical Symptoms

Treatment for Low Testosterone

About one-half of XXY males' chromosomes have low testosterone levels. These levels can be raised by taking supplemental testosterone. Testosterone treatment can:
- Improve muscle mass
- Deepen the voice
- Promote growth of facial and body hair
- Help the reproductive organs to mature
- Build and maintain bone strength and help prevent osteoporosis in later years
- Produce a more masculine appearance, which can also help relieve anxiety and depression
- Increase focus and attention

There are various ways to take testosterone:
- Injections or shots, every 2 to 3 weeks
- Pills
- Through the skin, also called "transdermal;" current methods include wearing a testosterone patch or rubbing testosterone gel on the skin

Males taking testosterone treatment should work closely with an endocrinologist, a doctor who specializes in hormones and their functions, to ensure the best outcome from testosterone therapy.

Treatment for Enlarged Breasts

No approved drug treatment exists for this condition of overdeveloped breast tissue, termed gynecomastia. Some healthcare providers recommend surgery—called "mastectomy"—to remove or reduce the breasts of XXY males.

When adult men have breasts, they are at higher risk for breast cancer than other men and need to be checked for this condition regularly. The mastectomy lowers the risk of cancer and can reduce the social stress associated with XXY males having enlarged breasts.

Because it is a surgical procedure, mastectomy carries a variety of risks. XXY males who are thinking about mastectomy should discuss all the risks and benefits with their healthcare provider.

Treatment for Infertility

Between 95 percent and 99 percent of XXY men are infertile because they do not produce enough sperm to fertilize an egg naturally. But, sperm are found in more than 50 percent of men with KS.

Advances in assistive reproductive technology (ART) have made it possible for some men with KS to conceive. One type of ART, called "testicular sperm extraction with intracytoplasmic sperm injection" (TESE-ICSI), has shown success for XXY males. For this procedure, a surgeon removes sperm from the testes and places one sperm into an egg.

Like all ART, TESE-ICSI carries both risks and benefits. For instance, it is possible that the resulting child might have the XXY condition. In addition, the procedure is expensive and is often is not covered by health insurance plans. Importantly, there is no guarantee the procedure will work.

Recent studies suggest that collecting sperm from adolescent XXY males and freezing the sperm until later might result in more pregnancies during subsequent fertility treatments. This is because although XXY males may make some healthy sperm during puberty, this becomes more difficult as they leave adolescence and enter adulthood.

Treating Language and Learning Symptoms

Some, but not all, children with KS have language development and learning delays. They might be slow to learn to talk, read, and write, and they might have difficulty processing what they hear. But, various interventions, such as speech therapy and educational assistance, can help to reduce and even eliminate these difficulties. The earlier treatment begins, the better the outcomes.

Parents might need to bring these types of problems to the teacher's attention. Because these boys can be quiet and cooperative in the classroom, teachers may not notice the need for help.

Boys and men with KS can benefit by visiting therapists who are experts in areas such as coordination, social skills, and coping. XXY males might benefit from any or all of the following:

- **Physical therapists** design activities and exercises to build motor skills and strength and to improve muscle control, posture, and balance.
- **Occupational therapists** help build skills needed for daily functioning, such as social and play skills, interaction and conversation skills, and job or career skills that match interests and abilities.
- **Behavioral therapists** help with specific social skills, such as asking other kids to play and starting conversations. They can also teach productive ways of handling frustration, shyness, anger, and other emotions that can arise from feeling "different."
- **Mental-health therapists** or counselors help males with KS find ways to cope with feelings of sadness, depression, self-doubt, and low self-esteem. They can also help with substance abuse problems. These professionals can also help families deal with the emotions of having a son with KS.
- **Family therapists** provide counseling to a man with KS, his spouse, partner, or family. They can help identify relationship problems and help patients develop communication skills and understand other people's needs.

Parents of XXY males have also mentioned that taking part in physical activities at low-key levels, such as karate, swimming, tennis, and golf, were helpful in improving motor skills, coordination, and confidence.

With regard to education, some boys with KS will qualify to receive state-sponsored special needs services to address their developmental and learning symptoms. But, because these symptoms may be mild, many XXY males will not be eligible for these services. Families can contact a local school district official or special education coordinator to learn more about whether XXY males can receive the following free services:

- The Early Intervention Program for Infants and Toddlers with Disabilities (www2.ed.gov/programs/osepeip/legislation.html) is required by two national laws, the Individuals with Disabilities and Education Improvement Act (IDEIA) and the Individuals with Disabilities Education Act (IDEA). Every state operates special programs for children from birth to age three, helping them develop in areas such as behavior, development, communication, and social play.
- An Individualized Education Plan (IEP) (www2.ed.gov/programs/specediep/legislation.html) for school is created and administered by a team of people, starting with parents and including teachers and school psychologists. The team works together to design an IEP with specific academic, communication, motor, learning, functional, and socialization goals, based on the child's educational needs and specific symptoms.

Treating Social and Behavioral Symptoms

Many of the professionals and methods for treating learning and language symptoms of the XXY condition are similar to or the same as the ones used to address social and behavioral symptoms.

For instance, boys with KS may need help with social skills and interacting in groups. Occupational or behavioral therapists might be able to assist with these skills. Some school districts and health centers might also offer these types of skill-building programs or classes.

In adolescence, symptoms such as lack of body hair could make XXY males uncomfortable in school or other social settings, and this discomfort can lead to depression, substance abuse, and behavioral problems or "acting out." They might also have questions about their masculinity or gender identity. In these instances, consulting a psychologist, counselor, or psychiatrist may be helpful.

Contrary to research results released decades ago, current research shows that XXY males are no more likely than other males to have serious psychiatric disorders or to get into trouble with the law.

How Do Healthcare Providers Diagnose Klinefelter Syndrome?

The only way to confirm the presence of an extra chromosome is by a karyotype test. A healthcare provider will take a small blood or skin sample and send it to a laboratory, where a technician inspects the cells under a microscope to find the extra chromosome. A karyotype test shows the same results at any time in a person's life.

Tests for chromosome disorders, including KS, may be done before birth. To obtain tissue or liquid for this test, a pregnant woman undergoes chorionic villus sampling or amniocentesis. These types of prenatal testing carry a small risk for miscarriage and are not routinely conducted unless the woman has a family history of chromosomal disorders, has other medical problems, or is above 35 years of age.

Factors That Influence When Klinefelter Syndrome Is Diagnosed

Because symptoms can be mild, some males with KS are never diagnosed.

Several factors affect whether and when a diagnosis occurs:

- Few newborns and boys are tested for or diagnosed with KS.
  - Although newborns in the United States are screened for some conditions, they are not screened for XXY or other sex-chromosome differences.
  - In childhood, symptoms can be subtle and overlooked easily. Only about 1 in 10 males with KS is diagnosed before puberty.
  - Sometimes, visiting a healthcare provider will not produce a diagnosis. Some symptoms, such as delayed early speech, might be treated successfully without further testing for KS.
- Most XXY diagnoses occur at puberty or in adulthood.

- Puberty brings a surge in diagnoses as some males (or their parents) become concerned about slow testes growth or breast development and consult a healthcare provider.
- Many men are diagnosed for the first time in fertility clinics. Among men seeking help for infertility, about 15 percent have KS.

Is There a Cure for Klinefelter Syndrome?

Currently, there is no way to remove chromosomes from cells to "cure" the XXY condition.

But, many symptoms can be successfully treated, minimizing the impact the condition has on length and quality of life. Most adult XXY men have full independence and have friends, families, and normal social relationships. They live about as long as other men, on average.

CHAPTER 24

LEARNING DISABILITY IN GIRLS WITH TURNER SYNDROME

About This Chapter: Text beginning with the heading "What Is Turner Syndrome?" is excerpted from "Turner Syndrome," Genetics Home Reference (GHR), National Institutes of Health (NIH), October 2017; Text beginning with the heading "Is Turner Syndrome Considered a Disability?" is excerpted from "Turner Syndrome: Other FAQs," *Eunice Kennedy Shriver* National Institute of Child Health and Human Development (NICHD), December 1, 2016. Reviewed July 2020.

What Is Turner Syndrome?

Turner syndrome is a chromosomal condition that affects development in females. The most common feature of Turner syndrome is short stature, which becomes evident by about age five. An early loss of ovarian function (ovarian hypofunction or premature ovarian failure) is also very common. The ovaries develop normally at first, but egg cells (oocytes) usually die prematurely and most ovarian tissue degenerates before birth. Many affected girls do not undergo puberty unless they receive hormone therapy, and most are unable to conceive (infertile). A small percentage of females with Turner syndrome retain normal ovarian function through young adulthood.

About 30 percent of females with Turner syndrome have extra folds of skin on the neck (webbed neck), a low hairline at the back of the neck, puffiness or swelling (lymphedema) of the hands and feet, skeletal abnormalities, or kidney problems. One-third to one half of individuals with Turner syndrome are born with a heart defect, such as a narrowing of the large artery leaving the heart (coarctation of the aorta) or abnormalities of the valve that connects the aorta with the heart (the aortic valve). Complications associated with these heart defects can be life-threatening.

Most girls and women with Turner syndrome have normal intelligence. Developmental delays, nonverbal learning disabilities, and behavioral problems are possible, although these characteristics vary among affected individuals.

Frequency of Turner Syndrome

This condition occurs in about one in 2,500 newborn girls worldwide, but it is much more common among pregnancies that do not survive to term (miscarriages and stillbirths).

Causes of Turner Syndrome

Turner syndrome is related to the X chromosome, which is one of the two sex chromosomes. People typically have two sex chromosomes in each cell: females have two X chromosomes, while males have one X chromosome and one Y chromosome. Turner syndrome results when one normal X chromosome is present in a female's cells and the other sex chromosome is missing or structurally altered. The missing genetic material affects development before and after birth.

About half of individuals with Turner syndrome have monosomy X, which means each cell in the individual's body has only one copy of the X chromosome instead of the usual two sex chromosomes. Turner syndrome can also occur if one of the sex chromosomes is partially missing or rearranged rather than completely absent. Some women with Turner syndrome have a chromosomal change in only some of their cells, which is known as "mosaicism." Women with Turner syndrome caused by X chromosome mosaicism are said to have mosaic Turner syndrome.

Researchers have not determined which genes on the X chromosome are associated with most of the features of Turner syndrome. They have, however, identified one gene called "*SHOX*" that is important for bone development and growth. The loss of one copy of this gene likely causes short stature and skeletal abnormalities in women with Turner syndrome.

Inheritance Pattern of Turner Syndrome

Most cases of Turner syndrome are not inherited. When this condition results from monosomy X, the chromosomal abnormality occurs as a random event during the formation of reproductive cells (eggs and sperm) in the affected person's parent. An error in cell division called "nondisjunction" can result in reproductive cells with an abnormal number of chromosomes. For example, an egg or sperm cell may lose a sex chromosome as a result of nondisjunction. If one of these atypical reproductive cells contributes to the genetic makeup of a child, the child will have a single X chromosome in each cell and will be missing the other sex chromosome.

Mosaic Turner syndrome is also not inherited. In an affected individual, it occurs as a random event during cell division in early fetal development. As a result, some of an affected person's cells have the usual two sex chromosomes, and other cells have only one copy of the X chromosome. Other sex chromosome abnormalities are also possible in females with X chromosome mosaicism.

Rarely, Turner syndrome caused by a partial deletion of the X chromosome can be passed from one generation to the next.

Is Turner Syndrome Considered a Disability?

Turner syndrome is not considered a disability, although it can cause certain learning challenges, including problems learning mathematics and with memory. Most girls and women with Turner syndrome lead a normal, healthy, productive life with proper medical care.

Your Daughter Has Been Diagnosed with Turner Syndrome. Now What?

If your daughter has been diagnosed with Turner syndrome, you may be wondering what to expect as she grows up.

Will She Have Problems in School?

Some girls with Turner syndrome have difficulty with arithmetic, visual memory, and visio-spatial skills (such as determining the relative positions of objects in space). They may also have some trouble understanding nonverbal communication (body language, facial expression) and interacting with peers.

What Care Will She Need as She Grows Up?

Girls with Turner syndrome usually require care from a variety of specialists throughout their lives.

CHAPTER 25
47,XYY SYNDROME

About This Chapter: This chapter includes text excerpted from "47,XYY Syndrome," Genetic and Rare Diseases Information Center (GARD), National Center for Advancing Translational Sciences (NCATS), January 14, 2018.

47,XYY syndrome is a syndrome (group of signs and symptoms) that affects males. For some males with this syndrome, signs and symptoms are barely noticeable. For others, signs and symptoms may include learning disabilities, speech delay, low muscle tone (hypotonia), and being taller than expected.

47,XYY syndrome is caused by having an extra copy of the Y chromosome in every cell of the body. The syndrome is usually not inherited. Diagnosis can be made based on prenatal tests, or it may occur during childhood or adulthood if a male has signs or symptoms of the disease. Management may include special education as well as intervention or therapies for developmental delays.

Symptoms of 47,XYY Syndrome

The signs and symptoms of 47,XYY syndrome can range from barely noticeable to more severe. It is thought that some males with 47,XYY syndrome may never be diagnosed because the signs and symptoms may not be noticeable. For other males, signs and symptoms such as low muscle tone (hypotonia) and/or speech delay may begin in late infancy or early childhood. Some boys with 47,XYY syndrome may have difficulty in certain subjects in school such as reading and writing. However, boys with this syndrome do not typically have intellectual disability.

Other signs and symptoms of 47,XYY syndrome may include asthma, dental problems, and acne. Boys with the syndrome do not typically have physical features different from most people, but they may be taller than expected. These boys are not expected to have differences in the appearance of the sex organs (genitalia). Some males with 47,XYY syndrome have behavioral differences such as autism spectrum disorder (usually on the milder end) or attention deficit hyperactivity disorder (ADHD). Boys with 47,XYY syndrome are also at an increased risk to have anxiety or mood disorders.

Most boys with 47,XYY syndrome go through normal sexual development, and fertility is expected to be normal. However, some boys with the syndrome may develop testicular failure (when the testes cannot produce sperm or testosterone), which can lead to problems with fertility.

Cause of 47,XYY Syndrome

47,XYY syndrome is caused by having an extra copy of the Y chromosome in each cell of the body. The Y chromosome is one of the sex chromosomes, and the other sex chromosome is called the "X chromosome." Most people have two sex chromosomes, with girls having two X chromosomes, and boys having one X and one Y chromosome.

Boys with 47,XYY syndrome have one X chromosome and two Y chromosomes in each cell of the body. This typically happens due to a random event when a sperm cell is formed that causes the sperm cell to have two Y chromosomes. When a sperm that has two Y chromosomes fertilizes an egg (which has an X chromosome), the resulting baby will be a male with two Y chromosomes and one X chromosome. It is also possible that a similar random event could occur very early in an embryo's development. This can produce a boy who has some cells that have two sex chromosomes and some cells that have an extra Y chromosome.

It is not fully understood why an extra copy of the Y chromosome causes the features associated with 47,XYY syndrome. It is thought that the tall stature seen in some males with the syndrome is caused by having an extra copy of a gene that is located on the sex chromosomes called the "SHOX" gene. This gene provides instructions to the body to control growth of the bones. People who have an extra copy of the Y chromosome also have an extra copy of the SHOX gene, which could explain why they may be taller than expected. Another gene that is thought to cause the signs and symptoms of 47,XYY syndrome is called "NLGN4Y." This gene is located on the Y chromosome and provides instructions to the body that helps form connections between the cells in the brain. It is thought that having an extra copy of this gene may cause the learning problems associated with 47,XYY syndrome.

Inheritance of 47,XYY Syndrome

47,XYY syndrome is usually not inherited from a parent. Instead, it is typically caused by a random event that happens during the formation of a sperm cell before conception (when the sperm fertilizes the egg). Even though this random event occurs in the sperm cell of the father of a person with 47,XYY syndrome, the syndrome is not inherited from the father because the father himself typically does not have the syndrome.

It is uncommon for more than one person in a family to have 47,XYY syndrome. If a couple has a child with 47,XYY syndrome, the chances for the couple or family members to have another child with the syndrome are not increased. Men who have 47,XYY syndrome themselves are also not thought to be at an increased risk to have a child with chromosome differences. Some sperm cells of a man with 47,XYY syndrome will have an extra Y chromosome. However, it is thought that these cells are less likely to be able to survive to fertilize an egg. Therefore, the chances for a man with 47,XYY syndrome to have a child with a sex chromosome abnormality are not thought to be increased.

People with questions about the chance to have a child with a chromosome abnormality are encouraged to speak with a genetic counselor or other genetics professional.

Diagnosis of 47,XYY Syndrome

47,XYY syndrome may be suspected when a doctor observes signs and symptoms that can be associated with the syndrome such as low muscle tone (hypotonia), speech delay, or learning problems in school. A doctor may then order testing to see if there is a genetic explanation for the signs and symptoms. Tests that may be ordered include:

- **Karyotype.** A test that is used to view all the chromosomes in a cell.
- **Chromosomal microarray.** A test that looks for extra or missing chromosomes or pieces of chromosomes.

In some cases, 47,XYY syndrome may be suspected prenatally based on routine screening tests. A diagnosis can be confirmed with prenatal tests such as an amniocentesis or chorionic villus sampling (CVS).

It is thought that some people who have 47,XYY syndrome are never diagnosed because they do not have severe signs or symptoms of the syndrome.

Treatment of 47,XYY Syndrome

The signs and symptoms of 47,XYY syndrome can be managed with a variety of therapies. Occupational therapy may be recommended for infants and young boys who have low muscle tone (hypotonia), and speech therapy may be recommended for boys who have speech delay. Boys with 47,XYY syndrome may be in special education at school, or they may have extra help in some classes.

Other management options for boys with 47,XYY syndrome may include behavioral therapy or medications for boys with ADHD or behavioral problems. If autism spectrum disorder is present, applied behavioral analysis (ABA) therapy may be recommended. In some cases, hormonal therapy may be used.

Prognosis of 47,XYY Syndrome

The long-term outlook for people with 47,XYY is typically good. Boys with this syndrome can do well both in school and in building social relationships. Men with 47,XYY syndrome can also have successful careers and families of their own. Therapies and other management for the syndrome can be important in allowing affected males to reach their full potentials.

CHAPTER 26
AARSKOG-SCOTT SYNDROME

About This Chapter: This chapter includes text excerpted from "Aarskog-Scott Syndrome," Genetics Home Reference (GHR), National Institutes of Health (NIH), May 26, 2020.

Aarskog-Scott syndrome is a genetic disorder that affects the development of many parts of the body. This condition mainly affects males, although females may have mild features of the syndrome.

People with Aarskog-Scott syndrome often have distinctive facial features, such as widely spaced eyes (hypertelorism), a small nose, a long area between the nose and mouth (philtrum), and a widow's peak hairline. They frequently have mild-to-moderate short stature during childhood, but their growth usually catches up with that of their peers during puberty. Hand abnormalities are common in this syndrome and include short fingers (brachydactyly), curved pinky fingers (fifth finger clinodactyly), webbing of the skin between some fingers (cutaneous syndactyly), and a single crease across the palm. Other abnormalities in people with Aarskog-Scott syndrome include heart defects and a split in the upper lip (cleft lip) with or without an opening in the roof of the mouth (cleft palate).

Most males with Aarskog-Scott syndrome have a shawl scrotum, in which the scrotum surrounds the penis instead of hanging below. Less often, they have undescended testes (cryptorchidism) or a soft out-pouching around the belly-button (umbilical hernia) or in the lower abdomen (inguinal hernia).

The intellectual development of people with Aarskog-Scott syndrome varies widely. Some may have mild learning and behavior problems, while others have normal intelligence. In rare cases, severe intellectual disability has been reported.

Frequency of Aarskog-Scott Syndrome

Aarskog-Scott syndrome is believed to be a rare disorder; however, its prevalence is unknown because mildly affected people may not be diagnosed.

Cause of Aarskog-Scott Syndrome

Mutations in the *FGD1* gene are the only known genetic cause of Aarskog-Scott syndrome. The *FGD1* gene provides instructions for making a protein that turns on (activates) another protein called "Cdc42," which transmits signals that are important for various aspects of development before and after birth.

Mutations in the *FGD1* gene lead to the production of an abnormally functioning protein. These mutations disrupt Cdc42 signaling, leading to the wide variety of abnormalities that occur in people with Aarskog-Scott syndrome.

Only about 20 percent of people with this disorder have identifiable mutations in the *FGD1* gene. The cause of Aarskog-Scott syndrome in other affected individuals is unknown.

Inheritance Pattern of Aarskog-Scott Syndrome

When caused by *FGD1* gene mutations, Aarskog-Scott syndrome is inherited in an X-linked recessive pattern. The *FGD1* gene is located on the X chromosome, which is one of the two sex chromosomes. In males (who have only one X chromosome), one altered copy of the gene in each cell is sufficient to cause the condition. In females (who have two X chromosomes), a mutation would have to occur in both copies of the gene to cause Aarskog-Scott syndrome. Because it is unlikely that females will have two altered copies of this gene, males are affected by X-linked recessive disorders much more frequently than females. Females who carry one altered copy of the *FGD1* gene may show mild signs of the condition, such as hypertelorism, short stature, or a widow's peak hairline. A characteristic of X-linked inheritance is that fathers cannot pass X-linked traits to their sons. Evidence suggests that Aarskog-Scott syndrome is inherited in an autosomal dominant or autosomal recessive pattern in some families, although the genetic cause of these cases is unknown. In autosomal dominant inheritance, one copy of the altered gene in each cell is sufficient to cause the disorder. In autosomal recessive inheritance, both copies of the gene in each cell have mutations. The parents of an individual with an autosomal recessive condition each carry one copy of the mutated gene, but they typically do not show signs and symptoms of the condition.

CHAPTER 27
SMITH-KINGSMORE SYNDROME

About This Chapter: This chapter includes text excerpted from "Smith-Kingsmore Syndrome," Genetics Home Reference (GHR), National Institutes of Health (NIH), May 26, 2020.

Smith-Kingsmore syndrome is a neurological disorder characterized by a head that is larger than normal (macrocephaly), intellectual disability, and seizures. In some people with this condition, the ability to speak is delayed or never develops. Some children with Smith-Kingsmore syndrome have features of a behavioral condition called "attention deficit hyperactivity disorder" (ADHD) or "autism spectrum disorder," which is characterized by impaired communication and social interaction. Structural brain abnormalities may also be present in affected individuals. For example, one or both sides of the brain may be enlarged (hemimegalencephaly or megalencephaly) or have too many ridges on the surface (polymicrogyria), or the fluid-filled spaces near the center of the brain (ventricles) may be bigger than normal (ventriculomegaly).

Many people with Smith-Kingsmore syndrome have unusual facial features, such as a triangular face with a pointed chin, a protruding forehead (frontal bossing), widely spaced eyes (hypertelorism) with outside corners that point downward (downslanting palpebral fissures), a flat nasal bridge, or a long space between the nose and upper lip (long philtrum). However, not everyone with Smith-Kingsmore syndrome has distinctive facial features.

Frequency of Smith-Kingsmore Syndrome
Smith-Kingsmore syndrome is a rare condition with an unknown prevalence.

Cause of Smith-Kingsmore Syndrome
Mutations in a gene called "MTOR" cause Smith-Kingsmore syndrome. The protein produced from this gene, called "mTOR," is a key piece of two groups of proteins, known as "mTOR complex 1" (mTORC1) and "mTOR complex2" (mTORC2). These two complexes relay signals inside cells that regulate protein production and control several cellular processes, including growth, division, and survival. This mTOR signaling

is especially important for growth and development of the brain, and it plays a role in a process called "synaptic plasticity," which is the ability of the connections between nerve cells (synapses) to change and adapt over time in response to experience. Synaptic plasticity is critical for learning and memory.

MTOR gene mutations that cause Smith-Kingsmore syndrome increase the activity of the mTOR protein and, consequently, mTOR signaling. As a result, protein production normally regulated by these complexes is uncontrolled, which impacts cell growth and division and other cellular processes. Too much mTOR signaling in brain cells disrupts brain growth and development and synaptic plasticity, leading to macrocephaly, intellectual disability, seizures, and other neurological problems in people with Smith-Kingsmore syndrome. Excessive mTOR signaling in other parts of the body likely underlies the unusual facial features and other less common signs and symptoms of the condition. It is unclear why the brain is particularly affected in people with Smith-Kingsmore syndrome.

Inheritance Pattern of Smith-Kingsmore Syndrome

Smith-Kingsmore syndrome follows an autosomal dominant inheritance pattern, which means one copy of the altered gene in each cell is sufficient to cause the disorder. Most cases result from new (de novo) mutations in the gene that occur during the formation of reproductive cells (eggs or sperm) in an affected individual's parent or in early embryonic development. Rarely, people with Smith-Kingsmore syndrome inherit the altered gene from an unaffected parent who has an *MTOR* gene mutation only in their sperm or egg cells. This phenomenon is called "germline mosaicism."

CHAPTER 28
TRIPLE X SYNDROME

About This Chapter: This chapter includes text excerpted from "Triple X Syndrome," Genetics Home Reference (GHR), National Institutes of Health (NIH), May 26, 2020.

Triple X syndrome, also called "trisomy X" or "47,XXX," is characterized by the presence of an additional X chromosome in each of a female's cells. Although females with this condition may be taller than average, this chromosomal change typically causes no unusual physical features. Most females with triple X syndrome have normal sexual development and are able to conceive children.

Triple X syndrome is associated with an increased risk of learning disabilities and delayed development of speech and language skills. Delayed development of motor skills (such as sitting and walking), weak muscle tone (hypotonia), and behavioral and emotional difficulties are also possible, but these characteristics vary widely among affected girls and women. Seizures or kidney abnormalities occur in about 10 percent of affected females.

Frequency of Triple X Syndrome

This condition occurs in about 1 in 1,000 newborn girls. 5 to 10 girls with triple X syndrome are born in the United States each day.

Causes of Triple X Syndrome

People normally have 46 chromosomes in each cell. Two of the 46 chromosomes, known as "X" and "Y," are called "sex chromosomes" because they help determine whether a person will develop male or female sex characteristics. Females typically have two X chromosomes (46,XX), and males have one X chromosome and one Y chromosome (46,XY).

Triple X syndrome results from an extra copy of the X chromosome in each of a female's cells. As a result of the extra X chromosome, each cell has a total of 47 chromosomes (47,XXX) instead of the usual 46. An extra copy of the X chromosome is associated with tall stature, learning problems, and other features in some girls and women.

Some females with triple X syndrome have an extra X chromosome in only some of their cells. This phenomenon is called "46,XX/47,XXX mosaicism."

Inheritance Pattern of Triple X Syndrome

Most cases of triple X syndrome are not inherited. The chromosomal change usually occurs as a random event during the formation of reproductive cells (eggs and sperm). An error in cell division called "nondisjunction" can result in reproductive cells with an abnormal number of chromosomes. For example, an egg or sperm cell may gain an extra copy of the X chromosome as a result of nondisjunction. If one of these atypical reproductive cells contributes to the genetic makeup of a child, the child will have an extra X chromosome in each of the body's cells.

46,XX/47,XXX mosaicism is also not inherited. It occurs as a random event during cell division in early embryonic development. As a result, some of an affected person's cells have two X chromosomes (46,XX), and other cells have three X chromosomes (47,XXX).

PART 4 | OTHER DISABILITIES AND CHRONIC CONDITIONS THAT IMPACT LEARNING

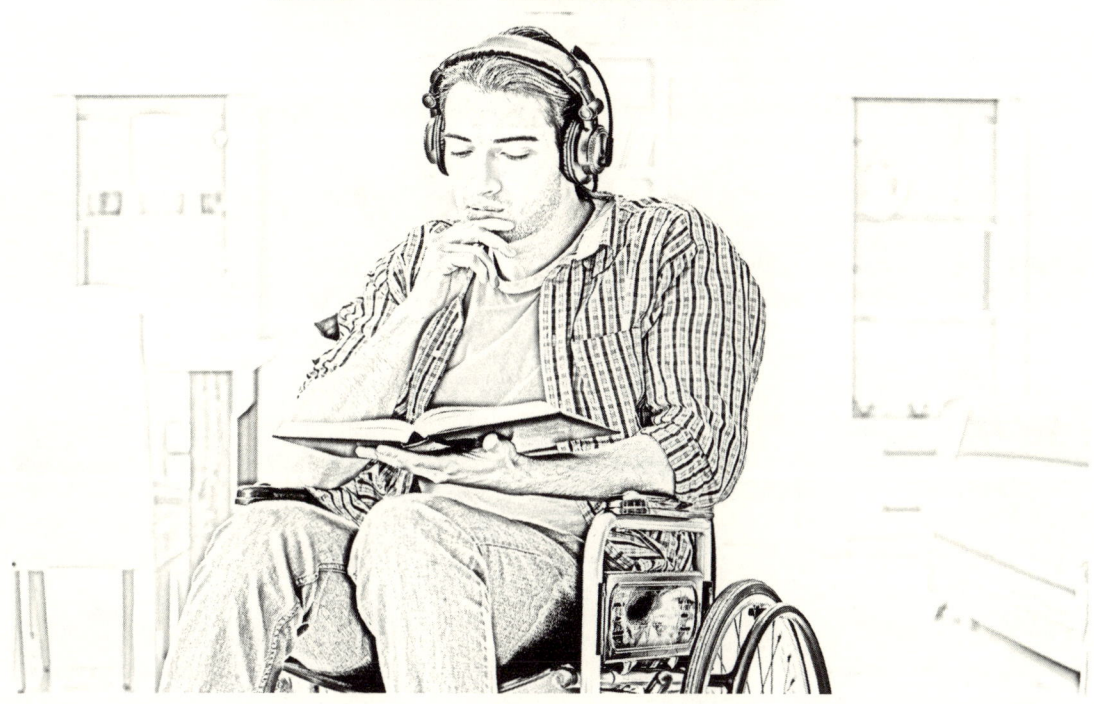

CHAPTER 29
BIPOLAR DISORDER AND LEARNING DISORDERS

About This Chapter: This chapter includes text excerpted from "Bipolar Disorder and Learning Disorders," National Institute of Mental Health (NIMH), March 12, 2020.

What Is Bipolar Disorder?

Bipolar disorder is a mental disorder that causes people to experience noticeable, sometimes extreme, changes in mood and behavior. Sometimes children with bipolar disorder feel very happy or "up" and are much more energetic and active than usual. This is called a "manic episode." Sometimes children with bipolar disorder feel very sad or "down" and are much less active than usual. This is called a "depressive episode."

Bipolar disorder, which used to be called "manic-depressive illness" or "manic depression," is not the same as the normal ups and downs every child goes through. The mood changes in bipolar disorder are more extreme, often unprovoked, and accompanied by changes in sleep, energy level, and the ability to think clearly. Bipolar symptoms can make it hard for young people to perform well in school or to get along with friends and family members. Some children and teens with bipolar disorder may try to hurt themselves or attempt suicide.

Does your child go through extreme changes in mood and behavior? Does your child get much more excited or much more irritable than other kids? Do you notice that your child goes through cycles of extreme highs and lows more often than other children? Do these mood changes affect how your child acts at school or at home?

Some children and teens with these symptoms may have bipolar disorder, a brain disorder that causes unusual shifts in mood, energy, activity levels, and day-to-day functioning. With treatment, children and teens with bipolar disorder can get better over time.

Most people are diagnosed with bipolar disorder in adolescence or adulthood, but the symptoms can appear earlier in childhood. Bipolar disorder is often episodic, but it usually lasts a lifetime.

Signs and symptoms of bipolar disorder may overlap with symptoms of other disorders that are common in young people, such as attention deficit hyperactivity disorder (ADHD), conduct problems, major depression, and anxiety disorders. Diagnosing bipolar disorder can be complicated and requires a careful and thorough evaluation by a trained, experienced mental-health professional.

With treatment, children and teens with bipolar disorder can manage their symptoms and lead successful lives.

What Causes Bipolar Disorder

The exact causes of bipolar disorder are unknown, but several factors may contribute to the illness.

For example, researchers are beginning to uncover genetic mechanisms that are linked to bipolar disorder and other mental disorders. Research shows that people's chance of having bipolar disorder is higher if they have a close family member with the illness, which may be because they have the same genetic variations. However, just because one family member has bipolar disorder, it does not mean that other members of the family will have it. Many genes are involved in the disorder, and no single gene causes it.

Research also suggests that adversity, trauma, and stressful life events may increase the chances of developing bipolar disorder in people with a genetic risk of having the illness.

Some research studies have found differences in brain structure and function between people who have bipolar disorder and those who do not. Researchers are studying the disorder to learn more about its causes and effective treatments.

What Are the Symptoms of Bipolar Disorder?

Mood episodes in bipolar disorder include intense emotions along with significant changes in sleep habits, activity levels, thoughts, or behaviors. A person with bipolar disorder may have manic episodes, depressive episodes, or "mixed" episodes. A mixed episode has both manic and depressive symptoms. These mood episodes cause symptoms that often last for several days or weeks. During an episode, the symptoms last every day for most of the day.

These mood and activity changes are very different from the child's usual behavior and from the behavior of healthy children and teens.

Children and teens having a manic episode may:

- Show intense happiness or silliness for long periods of time
- Have a very short temper or seem extremely irritable
- Talk fast about a lot of different things

Learning Difficulties

Bipolar disorder is a mental-health disorder that affects thinking and memory. A child with comorbid syndromes is distractable, inattentive, anxious, or a perfectionist. Some children also face cognitive problems as a result of medications. Others will have trouble organizing and accomplishing tasks.

In short, children with bipolar disorder will have difficulty in concentrating. It is also hard for them to study especially when they have poor memory. This will complicate their learning and ability to fulfill syllabus demands.

- Have trouble sleeping, but not feel tired
- Have trouble staying focused, and experience racing thoughts
- Seems overly interested or involved in pleasurable, but risky activities
- Do risky or reckless things that show poor judgment

Children and teens having a depressive episode may:
- Feel frequent and unprovoked sadness
- Show increased irritability, anger, or hostility
- Complain a lot about pain, such as stomachaches and headaches
- Have a noticeable increase in the amount of sleep
- Have difficulty concentrating
- Feel hopeless and worthless
- Have difficulty communicating or maintaining relationships
- Eat too much or too little
- Have little energy and no interest in activities they usually enjoy
- Think about death, or have thoughts of suicide

Can Children and Teens with Bipolar Disorder Have Other Problems?

Young people with bipolar disorder can have several problems at the same time. These include:
- **Misuse of alcohol and drugs.** Young people with bipolar disorder are at risk of misusing alcohol or drugs.
- **Attention deficit hyperactivity disorder.** Children and teens who have both bipolar disorder and ADHD may have trouble staying focused.
- **Anxiety disorders.** Children and teens with bipolar disorder also may have an anxiety disorder.

Sometimes extreme behaviors go along with mood episodes. During manic episodes, young people with bipolar disorder may take extreme risks that they would not usually take or that could cause them harm or injury. During depressive episodes, some young people with bipolar disorder may think about running away from home or have thoughts of suicide.

How Is Bipolar Disorder Diagnosed?

A healthcare provider will ask questions about your child's mood, sleeping patterns, energy levels, and behavior. There are no blood tests or brain scans that can diagnose bipolar disorder. However, the healthcare provider may use tests to see if something other than bipolar disorder is causing your child's symptoms. Sometimes healthcare providers need to know about medical conditions in the family, such as depression or substance use.

Other disorders that have symptoms such as those of bipolar disorder, include ADHD, disruptive mood regulation disorder, oppositional defiant disorder, conduct disorder, and anxiety disorders. It also can be challenging to distinguish bipolar disorder from depression that occurs without mania, which is referred to as "major depression." A healthcare provider who specializes in working with children and teens can make a careful and complete evaluation of your child's symptoms to provide the right diagnosis.

How Is Bipolar Disorder Treated?

Children and teens can work with their healthcare provider to develop a treatment plan that will help them manage their symptoms and improve their quality of life. It is important to follow the treatment plan, even when your child is not currently experiencing a mood episode. Steady, dependable treatment works better than treatment that starts and stops.

Treatment options include:

- **Medication.** Several types of medication can help treat symptoms of bipolar disorder. Children respond to medications in different ways, so the right type of medication depends on the child. This means children may need to try different types of medication to see which one works best for them. Some children may need more than one type of medication because their symptoms are complex. Children should take the fewest number of medications and the smallest doses possible to help their symptoms. A good way to remember this is "start low, go slow." Medications can cause side effects. Always tell your child's healthcare provider about any problems with side effects. Do not stop giving your child medication without speaking to a healthcare provider. Stopping medication suddenly can be dangerous and can make bipolar symptoms worse.

- **Psychosocial therapy.** Different kinds of psychosocial therapy can help children and their families manage the symptoms of bipolar disorder. Therapies that are based on scientific research—including cognitive behavioral approaches and family-focused therapy—can provide support, education, and guidance to youth and their families. These therapies teach skills that can help people manage bipolar disorder, including skills for maintaining routines, enhancing emotion regulation, and improving social interactions.

What Can Children and Teens Expect from Treatment?

With treatment, children and teens with bipolar disorder can get better over time. Treatment is more effective when healthcare providers, parents, and young people work together.

Sometimes a child's symptoms may change, or disappear and then come back. When this happens, your child's healthcare provider may recommend changes to the treatment plan. Treatment can take time, but sticking with the treatment plan can help young people manage their symptoms and reduce the likelihood of future episodes.

Your child's healthcare provider may recommend keeping a daily life chart or mood chart to track your child's moods, behaviors, and sleep patterns. This may make it easier to track the illness and see whether treatment is working.

How Can You Help Your Child or Teen?

Help begins with the right diagnosis and treatment. Talk to your family healthcare provider about any symptoms you notice.

If your child has bipolar disorder, here are some basic things you can do:

- Be patient.
- Encourage your child to talk, and listen to your child carefully.
- Pay attention to your child's moods, and be alert to any major changes.
- Understand triggers, and learn strategies for managing intense emotions and irritability.
- Help your child have fun.
- Remember that treatment takes time: sticking with the treatment plan can help your child get better and stay better.
- Help your child understand that treatment can make life better.

How Does Bipolar Disorder Affect Caregivers and Families?

Caring for a child or teenager with bipolar disorder can be stressful for parents and families. Coping with a child's mood episodes and other problems—such as short tempers and risky behaviors—can challenge any caregiver.

It is important that caregivers take care of themselves, too. Find someone you can talk to or consult your healthcare provider about support groups. Finding support and strategies for managing stress can help you and your child.

Where Do You Go for Help?

If you are not sure where to get help, your doctor, pediatrician, or other family healthcare provider is a good place to start. A healthcare provider can refer you to a qualified mental-health professional, such as a psychiatrist or psychologist, who has experience treating bipolar disorder and can evaluate your child's symptoms.

You can learn more about getting help and finding a healthcare provider (www.nimh.nih.gov/health/find-help/index.shtml) on the National Institute of Mental

Health (NIMH) website. Hospital healthcare providers can help in an emergency. The Substance Abuse and Mental Health Services Administration (SAMHSA) has an online tool to help you find mental-health services in your area (findtreatment.samhsa.gov).

If You Know Someone Who Is in Crisis. What Do You Do?

If you know someone who might be thinking about hurting themselves or someone else, get help quickly.

- Do not leave the person alone.
- Call 911 or go to the nearest hospital emergency room.
- Call the toll-free National Suicide Prevention Lifeline at 800-273-TALK (800-273-8255) or the toll-free TTY number at 800-799-4TTY (800-799-4889). You also can text the Crisis Text Line (text HELLO to 741741) or go to the National Suicide Prevention Lifeline (suicidepreventionlifeline.org) website.

CHAPTER 30

CEREBRAL PALSY AND SPECIFIC LEARNING DISABILITIES

About This Chapter: This chapter includes text excerpted from "Cerebral Palsy: Hope through Research," National Institute of Neurological Disorders and Stroke (NINDS), March 30, 2020.

What Is Cerebral Palsy?

Cerebral palsy (CP) refers to a group of neurological disorders that appear in infancy or early childhood and permanently affect body movement and muscle coordination. Cerebral palsy is caused by damage to or abnormalities inside the developing brain that disrupt the brain's ability to control movement and maintain posture and balance. The term cerebral refers to "the brain;" palsy refers to "the loss or impairment of motor function."

Cerebral palsy affects the motor area of the brain's outer layer (called the "cerebral cortex"), the part of the brain that directs muscle movement.

In some cases, the cerebral motor cortex has not developed normally during fetal growth. In others, the damage is a result of injury to the brain either before, during, or after birth. In either case, the damage is not repairable and the disabilities that result are permanent.

Children with CP exhibit a wide variety of symptoms, including:

- Lack of muscle coordination when performing voluntary movements (ataxia)
- Stiff or tight muscles and exaggerated reflexes (spasticity)
- Weakness in one or more arm or leg
- Walking on the toes, a crouched gait, or a "scissored" gait
- Variations in muscle tone, either too stiff or too floppy
- Excessive drooling or difficulties swallowing or speaking
- Shaking (tremor) or random involuntary movements
- Delays in reaching motor skill milestones
- Difficulty with precise movements such as writing or buttoning a shirt

The symptoms of CP differ in type and severity from one person to the next, and may even change in an individual over time. Symptoms may vary greatly among individuals, depending on which parts of the brain have been injured. All people with cerebral palsy have problems with movement and posture, and some also have some level of intellectual disability, seizures, and abnormal physical sensations or perceptions, as well as other medical disorders. People with CP also may have impaired vision or hearing, and language and speech problems.

Cerebral palsy is the leading cause of childhood disabilities, but it does not always cause profound disabilities. While one child with severe CP might be unable to walk and need extensive, lifelong care, another child with mild CP might be only slightly awkward and require no special assistance. The disorder is not progressive, meaning it does not get worse over time. However, as the child gets older, certain symptoms may become more or less evident.

A study by the Centers for Disease Control and Prevention shows the average prevalence of cerebral palsy is 3.3 children per 1,000 live births.

There is no cure for cerebral palsy, but supportive treatments, medications, and surgery can help many individuals improve their motor skills and ability to communicate with the world.

What Are the Early Signs?

The signs of cerebral palsy usually appear in the early months of life, although specific diagnosis may be delayed until age two years or later. Infants with CP frequently have developmental delay, in which they are slow to reach developmental milestones such as learning to roll over, sit, crawl, or walk. Some infants with CP have abnormal muscle tone. Decreased muscle tone (hypotonia) can make them appear relaxed, even floppy. Increased muscle tone (hypertonia) can make them seem stiff or rigid. In some cases, an early period of hypotonia will progress to hypertonia after the first 2 to 3 months of life. Children with CP may also have unusual posture or favor one side of the body when they reach, crawl, or move. It is important to note that some children without CP also might have some of these signs.

Some early warning signs:

In a Baby Younger than Six Months of Age
- Her or his head lags when you pick her or him up while she or he is lying on her or his back
- She or he feels stiff
- She or he feels floppy
- When you pick her or him up, her or his legs get stiff and they cross or scissor

In a Baby Older than Six Months of Age
- She or he does not roll over in either direction

- She or he cannot bring her or his hands together
- She or he has difficulty bringing her or his hands to her or his mouth
- She or he reaches out with only one hand while keeping the other fisted

In a Baby Older than Ten Months of Age
- She or he crawls in a lopsided manner, pushing off with one hand and leg while dragging the opposite hand and leg
- She or he cannot stand holding onto support

What Causes Cerebral Palsy

Cerebral palsy is caused by abnormal development of part of the brain or by damage to parts of the brain that control movement. This damage can occur before, during, or shortly after birth. The majority of children have congenital cerebral palsy CP (i.e., they were born with it), although it may not be detected until months or years later. A small number of children have acquired cerebral palsy, which means the disorder begins after birth. Some causes of acquired cerebral palsy include brain damage in the first few months or years of life, brain infections such as bacterial meningitis or viral encephalitis, problems with blood flow to the brain, or head injury from a motor vehicle accident, a fall, or child abuse.

In many cases, the cause of cerebral palsy is unknown. Possible causes include genetic abnormalities, congenital brain malformations, maternal infections or fevers, or fetal injury, for example. The following types of brain damage may cause its characteristic symptoms:

- **Damage to the white matter of the brain (Periventricular leukomalacia, or PVL).** The white matter of the brain is responsible for transmitting signals inside the brain and to the rest of the body. Damage from PVL looks like tiny holes in the white matter of an infant's brain. These gaps in brain tissue interfere with the normal transmission of signals. Researchers have identified a period of selective vulnerability in the developing fetal brain, a period of time between 26 and 34 weeks of gestation, in which periventricular white matter is particularly sensitive to insults and injury.
- **Abnormal development of the brain (Cerebral dysgenesis).** Any interruption of the normal process of brain growth during fetal development can cause brain malformations that interfere with the transmission of brain signals. Mutations in the genes that control brain development during this early period can keep the brain from developing normally. Infections, fevers, trauma, or other conditions that cause unhealthy conditions in the womb also put an unborn baby's nervous system at risk.
- **Bleeding in the brain (Intracranial hemorrhage).** Bleeding inside the brain from blocked or broken blood vessels is commonly caused by fetal

stroke. Some babies suffer a stroke while still in the womb because of blood clots in the placenta that block blood flow in the brain. Other types of fetal stroke are caused by malformed or weak blood vessels in the brain or by blood-clotting abnormalities. Maternal high blood pressure (hypertension) is a common medical disorder during pregnancy and is more common in babies with fetal stroke. Maternal infection, especially pelvic inflammatory disease, has also been shown to increase the risk of fetal stroke.

- **Severe lack of oxygen in the brain (Asphyxia).** A lack of oxygen in the brain caused by an interruption in breathing or poor oxygen supply, is common for a brief period of time in babies due to the stress of labor and delivery. If the supply of oxygen is cut off or reduced for lengthy periods, an infant can develop a type of brain damage called "hypoxic-ischemic encephalopathy," which destroys tissue in the cerebral motor cortex and other areas of the brain. This kind of damage can also be caused by severe maternal low blood pressure, rupture of the uterus, detachment of the placenta, or problems involving the umbilical cord, or severe trauma to the head during labor and delivery.

What Are the Risk Factors?

There are some medical conditions or events that can happen during pregnancy and delivery that may increase a baby's risk of being born with cerebral palsy. These risks include:

- **Low birth weight and premature birth.** Premature babies (born less than 37 weeks into pregnancy) and babies weighing less than 5 ½ pounds at birth have a much higher risk of developing cerebral palsy than full-term, heavier weight babies. Tiny babies born at very early gestational ages are especially at risk.

- **Multiple births.** Twins, triplets, and other multiple births—even those born at term—are linked to an increased risk of cerebral palsy. The death of a baby's twin or triplet further increases the risk.

- **Infections during pregnancy.** Infections such as toxoplasmosis, rubella (German measles), cytomegalovirus, and herpes, can infect the womb and placenta. Inflammation triggered by infection may then go on to damage the developing nervous system in an unborn baby. Maternal fever during pregnancy or delivery can also set off this kind of inflammatory response.

- **Blood type incompatibility between mother and child.** Rh incompatibility is a condition that develops when a mother's Rh blood type (either positive or negative) is different from the blood type of her baby. The mother's system does not tolerate the baby's different blood type and her body will begin to make antibodies that will attack and kill her baby's blood cells, which can cause brain damage.

- **Exposure to toxic substances.** Mothers who have been exposed to toxic substances during pregnancy, such as methyl mercury, are at a heightened risk of having a baby with cerebral palsy.
- **Mothers with thyroid abnormalities, intellectual disability, excess protein in the urine, or seizures.** Mothers with any of these conditions are slightly more likely to have a child with CP.

There are also medical conditions during labor and delivery, and immediately after delivery that act as warning signs for an increased risk of CP. However, most of these children will not develop CP. Warning signs include:

- **Breech presentation.** Babies with cerebral palsy are more likely to be in a breech position (feet first) instead of head first at the beginning of labor. Babies who are unusually floppy as fetuses are more likely to be born in the breech position.
- **Complicated labor and delivery.** A baby who has vascular or respiratory problems during labor and delivery may already have suffered brain damage or abnormalities.
- **Small for gestational age.** Babies born smaller than normal for their gestational age are at risk for cerebral palsy because of factors that kept them from growing naturally in the womb.
- **Low Apgar score.** The Apgar score is a numbered rating that reflects a newborn's physical health. Doctors periodically score a baby's heart rate, breathing, muscle tone, reflexes, and skin color during the first minutes after birth. A low score at 10 to 20 minutes after delivery is often considered an important sign of potential problems such as CP.
- **Jaundice.** More than 50 percent of newborns develop jaundice (a yellowing of the skin or whites of the eyes) after birth when bilirubin, a substance normally found in bile, builds up faster than their livers can break it down and pass it from the body. Severe, untreated jaundice can kill brain cells and can cause deafness and CP.
- **Seizures.** An infant who has seizures faces a higher risk of being diagnosed later in childhood with CP.

Can Cerebral Palsy Be Prevented?

Cerebral palsy related to genetic abnormalities cannot be prevented, but a few of the risk factors for congenital cerebral palsy can be managed or avoided. For example, rubella, or German measles, is preventable if women are vaccinated against the disease before becoming pregnant. Rh incompatibilities can also be managed early in pregnancy. Acquired cerebral palsy, often due to head injury, is often preventable using common safety tactics, such as using car seats for infants and toddlers.

What Are the Different Forms?

The specific forms of cerebral palsy are determined by the extent, type, and location of a child's abnormalities. Doctors classify CP according to the type of movement disorder involved—spastic (stiff muscles), athetoid (writhing movements), or ataxic (poor balance and coordination)—plus any additional symptoms, such as weakness (paresis) or paralysis (plegia). For example, hemiparesis (hemi = half) indicates that only one side of the body is weakened. Quadriplegia (quad = four) means all four limbs are affected.

Spastic cerebral palsy is the most common type of the disorder. People have stiff muscles and awkward movements. Forms of spastic cerebral palsy include:

- Spastic hemiplegia/hemiparesis typically affects the arm and hand on one side of the body, but it can also include the leg. Children with spastic hemiplegia generally walk later and on tip-toe because of tight heel tendons. The arm and leg of the affected side are frequently shorter and thinner. Some children will develop an abnormal curvature of the spine (scoliosis). A child with spastic hemiplegia may also have seizures. Speech will be delayed and, at best, may be competent, but intelligence is usually normal.
- Spastic diplegia/diparesis involves muscle stiffness that is predominantly in the legs and less severely affects the arms and face, although the hands may be clumsy. Tendon reflexes in the legs are hyperactive. Toes point up when the bottom of the foot is stimulated. Tightness in certain leg muscles makes the legs move like the arms of a scissor. Children may require a walker or leg braces. Intelligence and language skills are usually normal.
- Spastic quadriplegia/quadriparesis is the most severe form of cerebral palsy and is often associated with moderate-to-severe intellectual disability. It is caused by widespread damage to the brain or significant brain malformations. Children will often have severe stiffness in their limbs, but a floppy neck. They are rarely able to walk. Speaking and being understood are difficult. Seizures can be frequent and hard to control.

Dyskinetic cerebral palsy (also includes athetoid, choreoathetoid, and dystonic cerebral palsies) is characterized by slow and uncontrollable writhing or jerky movements of the hands, feet, arms, or legs. Hyperactivity in the muscles of the face and tongue makes some children grimace or drool. They find it difficult to sit straight or walk. Some children have problems hearing, controlling their breathing, and/or coordinating the muscle movements required for speaking. Intelligence is rarely affected in these forms of cerebral palsy.

Ataxic cerebral palsy affects balance and depth perception. Children with ataxic CP will often have poor coordination and walk unsteadily with a wide-based gait. They have difficulty with quick or precise movements, such as writing or buttoning a shirt, or a hard time controlling voluntary movement such as reaching from a book.

Mixed types of cerebral palsy refer to symptoms that do not correspond to any single type of CP but are a mix of types. For example, a child with mixed CP may have some muscles that are too tight and others that are too relaxed, creating a mix of stiffness and floppiness.

What Other Conditions Are Associated with Cerebral Palsy?

- **Intellectual disability.** Approximately 30 to 50 percent of individuals with CP will be intellectually impaired. Mental impairment is more common among those with spastic quadriplegia than in those with other types of cerebral palsy.
- **Seizure disorder.** As many as half of all children with CP have one or more seizures. Children with both cerebral palsy and epilepsy are more likely to have intellectual disability.
- **Delayed growth and development.** Children with moderate-to-severe CP, especially those with spastic quadriparesis, often lag behind in growth and development. In babies this lag usually takes the form of too little weight gain. In young children it can appear as abnormal shortness, and in teenagers it may appear as a combination of shortness and lack of sexual development. The muscles and limbs affected by CP tend to be smaller than normal, especially in children with spastic hemiplegia, whose limbs on the affected side of the body may not grow as quickly or as long as those on the normal side.
- **Spinal deformities and osteoarthritis.** Deformities of the spine—curvature (scoliosis), humpback (kyphosis), and saddle back (lordosis)—are associated with CP. Spinal deformities can make sitting, standing, and walking difficult and cause chronic back pain. Pressure on and misalignment of the joints may result in osteoporosis (a breakdown of cartilage in the joints and bone enlargement).
- **Impaired vision.** Many children with CP have strabismus, commonly called "cross eyes," which left untreated can lead to poor vision in one eye and can interfere with the ability to judge distance. Some children with CP have difficulty understanding and organizing visual information. Other children may have defective vision or blindness that blurs the normal field of vision in one or both eyes.
- **Hearing loss.** Impaired hearing is also more frequent among those with CP than in the general population. Some children have partial or complete hearing loss, particularly as the result of jaundice or lack of oxygen to the developing brain.
- **Speech and language disorders.** Speech and language disorders, such as difficulty forming words and speaking clearly, are present in more than a third of persons with CP. Poor speech impairs communication and is often interpreted as a sign of cognitive impairment, which can be very frustrating

to children with CP, especially the majority who have average to above-average intelligence.

- **Drooling.** Some individuals with CP drool because they have poor control of the muscles of the throat, mouth, and tongue.
- **Incontinence.** A possible complication of CP is incontinence, caused by poor control of the muscles that keep the bladder closed.
- **Abnormal sensations and perceptions.** Some individuals with CP experience pain or have difficulty feeling simple sensations, such as touch.
- **Learning difficulties.** Children with CP may have difficulty processing particular types of spatial and auditory information. Brain damage may affect the development of language and intellectual functioning.
- **Infections and long-term illnesses.** Many adults with CP have a higher risk of heart and lung disease, and pneumonia (often from inhaling bits of food into the lungs), than those without the disorder.
- **Contractures.** Muscles can become painfully fixed into abnormal positions, called "contractures," which can increase muscle spasticity and joint deformities in people with CP.
- **Malnutrition.** Swallowing, sucking, or feeding difficulties can make it difficult for many individuals with CP, particularly infants, to get proper nutrition and gain or maintain weight.
- **Dental problems.** Many children with CP are at risk of developing gum disease and cavities because of poor dental hygiene. Certain medications, such as seizure drugs, can exacerbate these problems.
- **Inactivity.** Childhood inactivity is magnified in children with CP due to impairment of the motor centers of the brain that produce and control voluntary movement. While children with CP may exhibit increased energy expenditure during activities of daily living, movement impairments make it difficult for them to participate in sports and other activities at a level of intensity sufficient to develop and maintain strength and fitness. Inactive adults with disability exhibit increased severity of disease and reduced overall health and well-being.

How Is Cerebral Palsy Diagnosed?

Most children with cerebral palsy are diagnosed during the first two years of life. But, if a child's symptoms are mild, it can be difficult for a doctor to make a reliable diagnosis before the age of four or five.

Doctors will order a series of tests to evaluate the child's motor skills. During regular visits, the doctor will monitor the child's development, growth, muscle tone, age-appropriate motor control, hearing and vision, posture, and coordination, in order to rule out other disorders that could cause similar symptoms. Although symptoms may change over time, CP is not progressive. If a child is continuously losing motor skills, the problem more likely is a condition other than CP—such as a genetic or muscle disease, metabolism disorder, or tumors in the nervous system.

Lab tests can identify other conditions that may cause symptoms similar to those associated with CP.

Neuroimaging techniques that allow doctors to look into the brain (such as an MRI scan) can detect abnormalities that indicate a potentially treatable movement disorder. Neuroimaging methods include:

- Cranial ultrasound uses high-frequency sound waves to produce pictures of the brains of young babies. It is used for high-risk premature infants because it is the least intrusive of the imaging techniques, although it is not as successful as computed tomography or magnetic resonance imaging at capturing subtle changes in white matter—the type of brain tissue that is damaged in CP.
- Computed tomography (CT) uses x-rays to create images that show the structure of the brain and the areas of damage.
- Magnetic resonance imaging (MRI) uses a computer, a magnetic field, and radio waves to create an anatomical picture of the brain's tissues and structures. MRI can show the location and type of damage and offers finer levels of details than CT.

Another test, an electroencephalogram, uses a series of electrodes that are either taped or temporarily pasted to the scalp to detect electrical activity in the brain. Changes in the normal electrical pattern may help to identify epilepsy.

Some metabolic disorders can masquerade as CP. Most of the childhood metabolic disorders have characteristic brain abnormalities or malformations that will show up on an MRI.

Other types of disorders can also be mistaken for CP or can cause specific types of CP. For example, coagulation disorders (which prevent blood from clotting or lead to excessive clotting) can cause prenatal or perinatal strokes that damage the brain and produce symptoms characteristic of CP, most commonly hemiparetic CP. Referrals to specialists such as a child neurologist, developmental pediatrician, ophthalmologist, or otologist aid in a more accurate diagnosis and help doctors develop a specific treatment plan.

How Is Cerebral Palsy Treated?

Cerebral palsy cannot be cured, but treatment will often improve a child's capabilities. Many children go on to enjoy near-normal adult lives if their disabilities are properly managed. In general, the earlier treatment begins, the better chance children have of overcoming developmental disabilities or learning new ways to accomplish the tasks that challenge them.

There is no standard therapy that works for every individual with cerebral palsy. Once the diagnosis is made, and the type of CP is determined, a team of healthcare professionals will work with a child and her or his parents to identify specific impairments and needs, and then develop an appropriate plan to tackle the core disabilities that affect the child's quality of life.

- Physical therapy, usually begun in the first few years of life or soon after the diagnosis is made, is a cornerstone of CP treatment. Specific sets of exercises (such as resistive, or strength training programs) and activities can maintain or improve muscle strength, balance, and motor skills, and prevent contractures. Special braces (called "orthotic devices") may be used to improve mobility and stretch spastic muscles.
- Occupational therapy focuses on optimizing upper body function, improving posture, and making the most of a child's mobility. Occupational therapists help individuals address new ways to meet everyday activities such as dressing, going to school, and participating in day-to-day activities.
- Recreation therapy encourages participation in art and cultural programs, sports, and other events that help an individual expand physical and cognitive skills and abilities. Parents of children who participate in recreational therapies usually notice an improvement in their child's speech, self-esteem, and emotional well-being.
- Speech and language therapy can improve a child's ability to speak, more clearly, help with swallowing disorders, and learn new ways to communicate—using sign language and/or special communication devices such as a computer with a voice synthesizer, or a special board covered with symbols of everyday objects and activities to which a child can point to indicate her or his wishes.
- Treatments for problems with eating and drooling are often necessary when children with CP have difficulty eating and drinking because they have little control over the muscles that move their mouth, jaw, and tongue. They are also at risk for breathing food or fluid into the lungs, as well as for malnutrition, recurrent lung infections, and progressive lung disease.

Drug Treatments

Oral medications such as diazepam, baclofen, dantrolene sodium, and tizanidine are usually used as the first line of treatment to relax stiff, contracted, or overactive muscles. Some drugs have some risk side effects such as drowsiness, changes in blood pressure, and risk of liver damage that require continuous monitoring. Oral medications are most appropriate for children who need only mild reduction in muscle tone or who have widespread spasticity.

- Botulinum toxin (BT-A), injected locally, has become a standard treatment for overactive muscles in children with spastic movement disorders such as CP. BT-A relax contracted muscles by keeping nerve cells from over-activating muscle. The relaxing effect of a BT-A injection lasts approximately three months. Undesirable side effects are mild and short-lived, consisting of pain upon injection and occasionally mild flu-like symptoms. BT-A injections are most effective when followed by a stretching program including physical therapy and splinting. BT-A injections work best for children who have some control over their motor movements and have a limited number of muscles to treat, none of which is fixed or rigid.

- Intrathecal baclofen therapy uses an implantable pump to deliver baclofen, a muscle relaxant, into the fluid surrounding the spinal cord. Baclofen decreases the excitability of nerve cells in the spinal cord, which then reduces muscle spasticity throughout the body. The pump can be adjusted if muscle tone is worse at certain times of the day or night. The baclofen pump is most appropriate for individuals with chronic, severe stiffness or uncontrolled muscle movement throughout the body.

Surgery

Orthopedic surgery is often recommended when spasticity and stiffness are severe enough to make walking and moving about difficult or painful. For many people with CP, improving the appearance of how they walk—their gait—is also important. Surgeons can lengthen muscles and tendons that are proportionately too short, which can improve mobility and lessen pain. Tendon surgery may help the symptoms for some children with CP, but could also have negative long-term consequences. Orthopedic surgeries may be staggered at times appropriate to a child's age and level of motor development. Surgery can also correct or greatly improve spinal deformities in people with CP. Surgery may not be indicated for all gait abnormalities and the surgeon may request a quantitative gait analysis before surgery.

Surgery to cut nerves. Selective dorsal rhizotomy (SDR) is a surgical procedure recommended for cases of severe spasticity when all of the more conservative treatments—physical therapy, oral medications, and intrathecal baclofen—have failed to reduce spasticity or chronic pain. A surgeon locates and selectively severs overactivated nerves at the base of the spinal column. SDR is most commonly used to relax muscles and decrease chronic pain in one or both of the lower or upper limbs. It is also sometimes used to correct an overactive bladder. Potential side effects include sensory loss, numbness, or uncomfortable sensations in limb areas once supplied by the severed nerve.

Assistive Devices

Assistive devices are devices such as computers, computer software, voice synthesizers, and picture books that can greatly help some individuals with CP improve communication skills. Other devices around the home or workplace make it easier for people with CP to adapt to activities of daily living.

Orthotic devices help to compensate for muscle imbalance and increase independent mobility. Braces and splints use external force to correct muscle abnormalities and improve function such as sitting or walking. Other orthotics help stretch muscles or the positioning of a joint. Braces, wedges, special chairs, and other devices can help people sit more comfortably and make it easier to perform daily functions. Wheelchairs, rolling walkers, and powered scooters can help individuals who are not independently mobile. Vision aids include glasses, magnifiers, and large-print books and computer typeface. Some individuals with CP may need surgery to correct vision problems. Hearing aids and telephone amplifiers may help people hear more clearly.

Complementary and Alternative Therapies

Many children and adolescents with CP use some form of complementary or alternative medicine. Controlled clinical trials involving some of the therapies have been inconclusive or showed no benefit and the therapies have not been accepted in mainstream clinical practice. Although there are anecdotal reports of some benefits in some children with CP, these therapies have not been approved by the U.S. Food and Drug Administration for the treatment of CP. Such therapies include hyperbaric oxygen therapy, special clothing worn during resistance exercise training, certain forms of electrical stimulation, assisting children in completing certain motions several times a day, and specialized learning strategies. Also, dietary supplements, including herbal products, may interact with other products or medications a child with CP may be taking or have unwanted side effects on their own. Families of children with CP should discuss all therapies with their doctor.

Stem cell therapy is being investigated as a treatment for cerebral palsy, but research is in early stages and large-scale clinical trials are needed to learn if stem cell therapy is safe and effective in humans. Stem cells are capable of becoming other cell types in the body. Scientists are hopeful that stem cells may be able to repair damaged nerves and brain tissues. Studies in the United States are examining the safety and tolerability of umbilical cord blood stem cell infusion in children with CP.

CHAPTER 31
EPILEPSY AND LEARNING DISABILITIES

About This Chapter: This chapter includes text excerpted from "Epilepsy in Schools," Centers for Disease Control and Prevention (CDC), May 29, 2019.

Epilepsy is a common disorder of the brain that causes recurring seizures. Epilepsy affects people of all ages, but children and older adults are more likely to have epilepsy. Seizures are the main sign of epilepsy and most people can control this with treatment. Some seizures can look like staring spells while other seizures can cause a person to collapse, stiffen or shake, and become unaware of what is going on around them. Many times the cause is unknown.

Picture a school with 1,000 students—that means about six students would have epilepsy. For many children, epilepsy is easily controlled with medication and they can do what all the other kids can do, and perform as well academically. For others, it can be more challenging.

Compared with students with other health concerns, the Centers for Disease Control and Prevention (CDC) study shows that students aged 6–17 years with epilepsy were more likely to miss 11 or more days of school in the past year. Also, students with epilepsy were more likely to have difficulties in school, use special education services, and have activity limitations such as less participation in sports or clubs compared with students with other medical conditions.

Managing Epilepsy at School

Managing epilepsy while at school may involve:

- Educating the school nurse, teachers, staff, and students about epilepsy and its treatment, seizure first aid, and possible stigma associated with epilepsy
- Following the seizure action plan and administering first aid (including the use of rescue medications)
- Understanding the importance of medication adherence and supporting students who take daily medications

Managing Epilepsy Well Checklist

Epilepsy can get in the way of life, mostly when seizures keep happening. You can learn how to manage your epilepsy to feel better and have a more active and full life. Practice these self-management strategies to better control your seizures and your health. Self-management is what you do to take care of yourself.

You manage your epilepsy well if you*:

- Know about your condition
- Take your seizure medicines as prescribed
- Check with your doctor before taking other medicines or supplements
- Keep a record of your seizures and seizure triggers to track patterns and learn how to avoid seizure triggers
- Get at least 7 to 8 hours of sleep each night
- Exercise regularly and safely each day
- Follow a well-balanced diet and keep a healthy weight
- Do not use tobacco, drink alcohol excessively, or abuse other substances
- Practice ways to lower stress
- Keep in touch with friends and family for support
- Talk to your doctor about health concerns
- Keep other health conditions in check
- Get help for emotional problems
- Use memory strategies to help with memory problems

How Well Are You Managing Your Epilepsy?

How many of the self-management strategies listed above do you already use to manage your epilepsy?

- **0 to 3:** You are on your way!
- **3 to 5:** Good job! Try to add a few more to your routine.
- **5 to 10:** Excellent! Keep up the good work!
- **10 or more:** You manage your epilepsy well!

Practicing self-management and still having seizures? Talk to your doctor about other treatment options.
*Modified from *Self-Management Goal Sheets. Agency for Healthcare Research and Quality (AHRQ); 2014.*
(Source: "Managing Epilepsy Well Checklist," Centers for Disease Control and Prevention (CDC))

- Helping students avoid seizure triggers, such as flashing lights, or other triggers identified in the seizure action plan
- Monitoring and addressing any related medical conditions, including mental-health concerns such as depression
- Providing case management services for students whose medical condition disrupts their school attendance or academic performance
- Referring students with uncontrolled seizures to medical services within the community or to the Epilepsy Foundation for more information
- Understanding the laws related to disability, medical conditions, and special education to ensure that children with epilepsy are able to access the free and appropriate education afforded to them under the law

- Monitoring student behavior to prevent bullying of students with epilepsy

What Is a Seizure Action Plan?

A Seizure Action Plan (www.epilepsy.com/learn/managing-your-epilepsy/seizure-action-plans) contains the essential information school staff may need to know in order to help a student who has seizures. It includes information on first aid, parent and healthcare provider contacts, and medications specifically for that child. Seizure Action Plans are an important tool that help parents and schools partner to keep children safe and healthy during the school day.

CHAPTER 32
AUTISTIC PEOPLE HAVE A LEARNING DISABILITY

About This Chapter: Text beginning with the heading "What Is Autism Spectrum Disorder?" is excerpted from "Autism Spectrum Disorder: Communication Problems in Children," National Institute on Deafness and Other Communication Disorders (NIDCD), April 13, 2020; Text under the heading "How Does Autism Spectrum Disorder Affects Teenagers and Adults" is excerpted from "Autism Spectrum Disorder in Teenagers and Adults," Centers for Disease Control and Prevention (CDC), March 26, 2020.

What Is Autism Spectrum Disorder?

Autism spectrum disorder (ASD) is a developmental disability that can cause significant social, communication, and behavioral challenges. The term "spectrum" refers to the wide range of symptoms, skills, and levels of impairment that people with ASD can have.

Autism spectrum disorder affects people in different ways and can range from mild-to-severe. People with ASD share some symptoms, such as difficulties with social interaction, but there are differences in when the symptoms start, how severe they are, the number of symptoms, and whether other problems are present. The symptoms and their severity can change over time.

The behavioral signs of ASD often appear early in development. Many children show symptoms by 12 months to 18 months of age or earlier.

Who Is Affected By Autism Spectrum Disorder?

Autism spectrum disorder affects people of every race, ethnic group, and socioeconomic background. It is four times more common among boys than among girls. The Centers for Disease Control and Prevention (CDC) estimates that about one in every 54 children in the United States has been identified as having ASD.

How Does Autism Spectrum Disorder Affect Communication?

The word "autism" has its origin in the Greek word "autos," which means "self." Children with ASD are often self-absorbed and seem to exist in a private world in which they have limited ability to successfully communicate and interact with others. Children with ASD may have difficulty developing language skills and understanding what others say to them. They also often have difficulty communicating nonverbally, such as through hand gestures, eye contact, and facial expressions.

The ability of children with ASD to communicate and use language depends on their intellectual and social development. Some children with ASD may not be able to communicate using speech or language, and some may have very limited speaking skills. Others may have rich vocabularies and be able to talk about specific subjects in great detail. Many have problems with the meaning and rhythm of words and sentences. They also may be unable to understand body language and the meanings of different vocal tones. Taken together, these difficulties affect the ability of children with ASD to interact with others, especially people their own age.

Below are some patterns of language use and behaviors that are often found in children with ASD.

- **Repetitive or rigid language.** Often, children with ASD who can speak will say things that have no meaning or that do not relate to the conversations they are having with others. For example, a child may count from one to five repeatedly amid a conversation that is not related to numbers. Or a child may continuously repeat words she or he has heard—a condition called "echolalia." Immediate echolalia occurs when the child repeats words someone has just said. For example, the child may respond to a question by asking the same question. In delayed echolalia, the child repeats words heard at an earlier time. The child may say "Do you want something to drink?" whenever she or he asks for a drink. Some children with ASD speak in a high-pitched or sing-song voice or use robot-like speech. Other children may use stock phrases to start a conversation. For example, a child may say, "My name is Tom," even when he talks with friends or family. Still, others may repeat what they hear on television programs or commercials.

- **Narrow interests and exceptional abilities.** Some children may be able to deliver an in-depth monologue about a topic that holds their interest, even though they may not be able to carry on a two-way conversation about the same topic. Others may have musical talents or an advanced ability to count and do math calculations. Approximately 10 percent of children with ASD show "savant" skills, or extremely high abilities in specific areas, such as memorization, calendar calculation, music, or math.

- **Uneven language development.** Many children with ASD develop some speech and language skills, but not to a normal level of ability, and their progress is usually uneven. For example, they may develop a strong vocabulary in a particular area of interest very quickly. Many children have good memories for information just heard or seen. Some may be able to read words before age five, but may not comprehend what they have read.

They often do not respond to the speech of others and may not respond to their own names. As a result, these children are sometimes mistakenly thought to have a hearing problem.

- **Poor nonverbal conversation skills.** Children with ASD are often unable to use gestures—such as pointing to an object—to give meaning to their speech. They often avoid eye contact, which can make them seem rude, uninterested, or inattentive. Without meaningful gestures or other nonverbal skills to enhance their oral language skills, many children with ASD become frustrated in their attempts to make their feelings, thoughts, and needs known. They may act out their frustrations through vocal outbursts or other inappropriate behaviors.

How Are the Speech and Language Problems of Autism Spectrum Disorder Treated?

If a doctor suspects a child has ASD or another developmental disability, she or he usually will refer the child to a variety of specialists, including a speech-language pathologist. This is a health professional trained to treat individuals with voice, speech, and language disorders. The speech-language pathologist will perform a comprehensive evaluation of the child's ability to communicate, and will design an appropriate treatment program. In addition, the speech-language pathologist might make a referral for a hearing test to make sure the child's hearing is normal.

Teaching children with ASD to improve their communication skills is essential for helping them reach their full potential. There are many different approaches, but the best treatment program begins early, during the preschool years, and is tailored to the child's age and interests. It should address both the child's behavior and communication skills and offer regular reinforcement of positive actions. Most children with ASD respond well to highly structured, specialized programs. Parents or primary caregivers, as well as other family members, should be involved in the treatment program so that it becomes part of the child's daily life.

For some younger children with ASD, improving speech and language skills is a realistic goal of treatment. Parents and caregivers can increase a child's chance of reaching this goal by paying attention to her or his language development early on. Just as toddlers learn to crawl before they walk, children first develop prelanguage skills before they begin to use words. These skills include using eye contact, gestures, body movements, imitation, and babbling and other vocalizations to help them communicate. Children who lack these skills may be evaluated and treated by a speech-language pathologist to prevent further developmental delays.

For slightly older children with ASD, communication training teaches basic speech and language skills, such as single words and phrases. Advanced training emphasizes the way language can serve a purpose, such as learning to hold a conversation with another person, which includes staying on topic and taking turns speaking.

Some children with ASD may never develop oral speech and language skills. For these children, the goal may be learning to communicate using gestures, such as sign language. For others, the goal may be to communicate by means of a symbol system in which pictures are used to convey thoughts. Symbol systems can range from picture boards or cards to sophisticated electronic devices that generate speech through the use of buttons to represent common items or actions.

How Does Autism Spectrum Disorder Affects Teenagers and Adults

A greater number of children identified with ASD has led to a growing interest in the transition to adolescence and adulthood. For most young people, including those with ASD, adolescence and young adulthood are filled with new challenges, responsibilities, and opportunities. However, research suggests fewer young people with ASD have the same opportunities as their peers without ASD.

- High rates of unemployment or under-employment
- Low participation in education beyond high school
- Majority continue to live with family members or relatives
- Limited opportunity for community or social activities—nearly 40 percent spend little or no time with friends

In addition, individuals with ASD may experience changes in their ASD symptoms, behaviors, and co-occurring health conditions during adolescence and young adulthood. These changes can affect their ability to function and participate in the community.

The Centers for Disease Control and Prevention's Work for Adults with Autism Spectrum Disorder

Planning for Service Needs

The CDC's most recent funding cycle for the Autism and Developmental Disabilities Monitoring (ADDM) Network (www.cdc.gov/ncbddd/autism/addm.html) includes support for five sites to follow up on 16-year-olds who had been identified with ASD by 8 years of age. This is a new activity for the ADDM Network and will provide valuable information on transition planning in special education services and potential service needs after high school.

Promoting Better Outcomes

The CDC's Study to Explore Early Development (SEED) (www.cdc.gov/ncbddd/autism/seed.html) began identifying children with ASD in the mid-2000s and these children are now beginning the transition from adolescence to adulthood. Through SEED Teen, the CDC is tracking the changes that occur during this transition period to learn about factors that may promote more successful transitions and better outcomes in young adults with ASD.

CHAPTER 33
LEARNING PROBLEMS IN CHILDHOOD CANCER

About This Chapter: This chapter includes text excerpted from "Late Effects of Treatment for Childhood Cancer (PDQ®)—Patient Version," National Cancer Institute (NCI), March 10, 2020.

Late Effects of Treatment That Affect the Brain and Spinal Cord May Cause Certain Health Problems

Childhood cancer survivors who received radiation, certain types of chemotherapy, or surgery to the brain or spinal cord have an increased risk of late effects to the brain and spinal cord and related health problems. These include the following:

- Headaches
- Loss of coordination and balance
- Dizziness
- Seizures
- Loss of the myelin sheath that covers nerve fibers in the brain
- Movement disorders that affect the legs and eyes or the ability to speak and swallow
- Nerve damage in the hands or feet
- Stroke. A second stroke may be more likely in survivors who received radiation to the brain, have a history of high blood pressure, or were older than 40 years when they had their first stroke.
- Daytime sleepiness
- Hydrocephalus
- Loss of bladder and/or bowel control
- Cavernomas (clusters of abnormal blood vessels)
- Back pain

Survivors may also have late effects that affect thinking, learning, memory, emotions, and behavior.

New ways of using more targeted and lower doses of radiation to the brain may lessen the risk of brain and spinal cord late effects.

Radiation to the Brain Increases the Risk of Brain and Spinal Cord Late Effects

The risk of health problems that affect the brain or spinal cord increases after treatment with the following:
- Radiation to the brain or spinal cord, especially high doses of radiation. This includes total-body irradiation given as part of a stem cell transplant.
- Intrathecal or intraventricular chemotherapy
- Chemotherapy with high-dose methotrexate or cytarabine that can cross the blood-brain barrier (protective lining around the brain). This includes high-dose chemotherapy given as part of a stem cell transplant.
- Surgery to remove a tumor on the brain or spinal cord
- When radiation to the brain and intrathecal chemotherapy are given at the same time, the risk of late effects is higher.

The following may also increase the risk of brain and spinal cord late effects in childhood brain tumor survivors:
- Being about 5 years old or younger at the time of treatment
- Being female
- Having hydrocephalus and a shunt placed to removed the extra fluid from the ventricles
- Having hearing loss
- Having cerebellar mutism following surgery to remove the brain tumor. Cerebellar mutism includes not being able to speak, loss of coordination

and balance, mood swings, being irritable, and having a high-pitched cry.
- Having a personal history of stroke
- Seizures

Central nervous system late effects are also affected by where the tumor has formed in the brain and spinal cord.

Possible Signs and Symptoms of Brain and Spinal Cord Late Effects Include Headaches, Loss of Coordination, and Seizures

These signs and symptoms may be caused by brain and spinal cord late effects or by other conditions:
- Headache that may go away after vomiting
- Seizures
- Loss of balance, lack of coordination, or trouble walking
- Trouble speaking or swallowing
- Trouble with having the eyes work together
- Numbness, tingling, or weakness in the hands or feet
- Being unable to bend the ankle to lift the foot up
- Sudden numbness or weakness of the face, arm, or leg (especially on one side of the body)
- Unusual sleepiness or change in activity level
- Unusual changes in personality or behavior
- A change in bowel habits or trouble urinating
- Increase in head size (in infants)
- Sudden confusion or trouble speaking or understanding speech
- Sudden trouble seeing with one or both eyes
- Sudden severe headache for no known reason

Other signs and symptoms include the following:
- Problems with memory
- Problems with paying attention
- Trouble with solving problems
- Trouble with organizing thoughts and tasks
- Slower ability to learn and use new information
- Trouble learning to read, write, or do math
- Trouble coordinating movement between the eyes, hands, and other muscles
- Delays in normal development
- Social withdrawal or trouble getting along with others
- Talk to your child's doctor if your child has any of these problems

Certain Tests and Procedures Are Used to Diagnose Health Problems in the Brain and Spinal Cord

These and other tests and procedures may be used to detect or diagnose brain and spinal cord late effects:

- **Physical exam and health history.** An exam of the body to check general signs of health, including checking for signs of disease, such as lumps or anything else that seems unusual. A history of the patient's health habits and past illnesses and treatments will also be taken.
- **Neurological exam.** A series of questions and tests to check the brain, spinal cord, and nerve function. The exam checks a person's mental status, coordination, and ability to walk normally, and how well the muscles, senses, and reflexes work. This may also be called a "neuro exam" or a "neurologic exam." In some cases, a more complete exam may be done by a neurologist or neurosurgeon.
- **Neuropsychological assessment.** A series of tests to examine the patient's mental processes and behavior. Areas that are checked usually include:
  - Knowing who and where you are and what day it is
  - Ability to learn and remember new information
  - Intelligence
  - Ability to solve problems
  - Use of spoken and written language
  - Eye-hand coordination
  - Ability to organize information and tasks

Talk to your child's doctor about whether your child needs to have tests and procedures to check for signs of brain and spinal cord late effects. If tests are needed, find out how often they should be done.

Survivors of Childhood Cancer May Have Anxiety and Depression Related to Their Cancer

Survivors of childhood cancer may have anxiety and depression related to physical changes, having pain, the way they look, or the fear of cancer coming back. These and other factors may cause problems with personal relationships, education, employment, and health, and cause thoughts of suicide. Survivors with these problems may be less likely to live on their own as adults.

Follow-up exams for childhood cancer survivors should include screening and treatment for possible psychological distress, such as anxiety, depression, and thoughts of suicide.

Some Childhood Cancer Survivors Have Posttraumatic Stress Disorder

Being diagnosed and treated for a life-threatening disease may be traumatic. This trauma may cause posttraumatic stress disorder (PTSD). PTSD is defined as having certain behaviors following a stressful event that involved death or the threat of death, serious injury, or a threat to oneself or others.

Posttraumatic stress disorder can affect cancer survivors in the following ways:

- Reliving the time they were diagnosed and treated for cancer, in nightmares or flashbacks, and thinking about it all the time
- Avoiding places, events, and people that remind them of the cancer experience

In general, childhood cancer survivors show low levels of PTSD, depending in part on the coping style of patients and their parents. Survivors who received radiation therapy to the head when younger than 4 years or survivors who received intensive treatment may be at higher risk of PTSD. Family problems, little or no social support from family or friends, and stress not related to the cancer may increase the chances of having PTSD.

Because avoiding places and persons connected to the cancer may be part of PTSD, survivors with PTSD may not get the medical treatment they need.

Adolescents Who Are Diagnosed with Cancer May Have Social Problems Later in Life

Adolescents who are diagnosed with cancer may reach fewer social milestones or reach them later in life than adolescents not diagnosed with cancer. Social milestones include having a first boyfriend or girlfriend, getting married, and having a child. They may also have trouble getting along with other people or feel like they are not liked by others their age.

Cancer survivors in this age group have reported being less satisfied with their health and their lives in general compared with others of the same age who did not have cancer. Adolescents and young adults who have survived cancer need special programs that give psychological, educational, and job support.

CHAPTER 34

DRUG ABUSE AND YOUR HIGH-SCHOOL GRADES

About This Chapter: This chapter includes text excerpted from "How Does Drug Use Affect Your High School Grades?" Just Think Twice, U.S. Drug Enforcement Administration (DEA), October 14, 2014. Reviewed July 2020.

Did you know that your brain develops until the age of 25? Anything that you do to disrupt this process—including substance—will affect how your brain develops.

During the brain's development stage, any type of trauma and/or changes in the brain's wiring could affect brain function. Drug use is one of the ways that can mess up the wiring. How?

According to the National Institute on Drug Abuse (NIDA), the brain relies on chemicals called "neurotransmitters" to get messages from one part of the brain to the other. Each neurotransmitter attaches to its own kind of receptor—like how a key fits into a lock. This allows messages to travel through the brain on the right path. When you use drugs, it interferes with the normal traffic patterns that the neurotransmitters use. The chemical structure in the drugs can imitate and fool the receptors, lock on to them and alter the activity of the nerve cells. This "alteration" can result in messages going in the wrong direction, and reset the way your brain should act or react.

Ultimately this affects the way your brain processes and retains information—and how you think, learn, remember, focus, and concentrate.

Research shows that there is a definite link between teen substance abuse and how well you do in school. Teens who abuse drugs have lower grades, a higher rate of absence from school and other activities, and an increased potential for dropping out of school.

Although we all know or hear stories about people who use drugs and still get great grades, this is not typical. Most people who use drugs regularly do not consistently do well in school.

Studies show that marijuana, for example, affects your attention, memory, and ability to learn. Its effects can last for days or weeks after the drug wears off. So, if you are smoking marijuana daily, you are not functioning at your best.

Students who smoke marijuana tend to get lower grades and are more likely to drop out of high school. One recent marijuana study showed that heavy marijuana use in your teen years and continued into adulthood can reduce your intelligence quotient (IQ) up to as much as eight points.

High school dropout rates have also risen as a result of substance abuse.

A study of teens in 12th grade (16–18 years of age) who dropped out of school before graduation are more likely than their peers to be users of cigarettes, alcohol, marijuana, and other illicit drugs.

Illicit drug use among dropouts was higher than for those in school (31.4% versus 18.2%). Dropouts were more likely to be current marijuana users than those in school (27.3 % versus 15.3 %) and nonmedical users of prescription drugs (9.5% versus 5.1%).

Teens who smoke, drink alcohol, binge drink, or use marijuana or other drugs are more likely than nonusers to drop out of school and less likely than nonusers to graduate from high school, attend college, or obtain a college degree. One study found that nearly one-third of school dropouts indicate that their use of alcohol or other drugs was an important contributor in their decision to leave school.

CHAPTER 35
CHILDHOOD LEAD POISONING

About This Chapter: This chapter includes text excerpted from "Childhood Lead Poisoning," Centers for Disease Control and Prevention (CDC), May 2005. Reviewed July 2020.

Approximately 310,000 Children in the United States aged one to five years have blood lead levels greater than 10 micrograms of lead per deciliter of blood, a level at which harmful health effects are known to occur.

Lead poisoning can affect nearly every system in the body. Because lead poisoning often occurs with no obvious symptoms, it frequently goes unrecognized. Lead poisoning can cause learning disabilities, behavioral problems, and, at very high levels, seizures, coma, and even death.

How Are Children Exposed to Lead?

The major source of lead exposure among children in the United States is lead-based paint and lead-contaminated dust found in deteriorating buildings. Lead-based paints were banned for use in housing in 1978. However, approximately 24 million housing units in the United States have deteriorated leaded paint and elevated levels of lead-contaminated house dust. More than four million of these dwellings are home to one or more young children.

Other sources of lead poisoning are related to:

- Home health remedies (azarcon and greta, which are used for upset stomach or indigestion; pay-loo-ah, which is used for rash or fever)
- Some imported candies (specifically those from Mexico)
- Imported toy jewelry
- Drinking water (lead pipes, solder, brass fixtures, and valves can all leach lead)
- Work (recycling or making automobile batteries)
- Hobbies (making stained-glass windows)

Who Is at Risk?

- Children under the age of six years because they are growing so rapidly and because they tend to put their hands or other objects into their mouths.
- Children from all social and economic levels can be affected by lead poisoning, although children living at or below the poverty line who live in older housing are at greatest risk.
- Children of some racial and ethnic groups and those living in older housing are disproportionately affected by lead. For example, three percent of black children compared to 1.3 percent of white children have elevated blood lead levels.

Can Lead Poisoning Be Prevented?

Lead poisoning is entirely preventable. The key is stopping children from coming into contact with lead and treating children who have been poisoned by lead.

- Lead hazards in a child's environment must be identified and removed safely.
- Parents, healthcare professionals, and the general public need education about lead poisoning and how to prevent it.
- Children who are at risk for lead poisoning need to be tested, and, if necessary, treated.

What Can Parents and the Public Do to Reduce Blood Lead Levels?

- Ask a doctor to test your child if you are concerned about your child being exposed to lead.
- Talk to your state or local health department about testing paint and dust from your home for lead if you live in a house or apartment built before 1978, especially if young children live with you or visit you.
- Damp-mop floors; damp-wipe surfaces; and frequently wash a child's hands, pacifiers, and toys to reduce exposure to lead.
- Avoid using home remedies (such as arzacon, greta, pay-loo-ah) and cosmetics (such as kohl, alkohl) that contain lead.
- At this time, children and pregnant women should not eat candies imported from Mexico.
- Use only cold water from the tap for drinking, cooking, and making baby formula. Hot water is more likely to contain higher levels of lead, and most of the lead in household water usually comes from the plumbing in your house, not from the local water supply.
- Take basic steps to decrease your exposure to lead (e.g., by showering and changing clothes after finishing the task) if you remodel buildings built before 1978 or if your work or hobbies involve working with lead-based products.

The Centers for Disease Control and Prevention's Role in Preventing Lead Poisoning

- The Centers for Disease Control and Prevention (CDC) provides technical and financial assistance to state and local childhood lead poisoning prevention programs. These programs are working to ensure that screening, lead-hazard reduction, new legislation, and other prevention mechanisms occur throughout the country.
- The CDC has established a national system to identify children with elevated blood lead levels.
- The CDC provides guidance for the proper care of children after they are identified as having elevated blood lead levels.
- The CDC provides national guidance and policy for the prevention of childhood lead poisoning.
- The CDC will continue to work with state and local areas to improve capacity and provide guidance.

CHAPTER 36

UNDERSTANDING TOURETTE SYNDROME AND ITS EFFECTS ON LEARNING

About This Chapter: This chapter includes text excerpted from "Tourette Syndrome (TS)—What Is Tourette Syndrome?" Centers for Disease Control and Prevention (CDC), May 23, 2019.

What Is Tourette Syndrome?

Tourette syndrome (TS) is a condition of the nervous system. TS causes people to have "tics."

Tics are sudden twitches, movements, or sounds that people do repeatedly. People who have tics cannot stop their body from doing these things. For example, a person might keep blinking over and over again. Or, a person might make a grunting sound unwillingly.

Having tics is a little bit like having hiccups. Even though you might not want to hiccup, your body does it anyway. Sometimes people can stop themselves from doing a certain tic for a while, but it is hard. Eventually the person has to do the tic.

Types of Tics

There are two types of tics—motor and vocal.

Motor Tics

Motor tics are movements of the body. Examples of motor tics include blinking, shrugging the shoulders, or jerking an arm.

Vocal Tics

Vocal tics are sounds that a person makes with her or his voice. Examples of vocal tics include humming, clearing the throat, or yelling out a word or phrase.

Tics can be either simple or complex.

Simple Tics

Simple tics involve just a few parts of the body. Examples of simple tics include squinting the eyes or sniffing.

Complex Tics

Complex tics usually involve several different parts of the body and can have a pattern. An example of a complex tic is bobbing the head while jerking an arm, and then umping up.

Symptoms of Tourette Syndrome

The main symptoms of TS are tics. Symptoms usually begin when a child is 5 to 10 years of age. The first symptoms often are motor tics that occur in the head and neck area. Tics usually are worse during times that are stressful or exciting. They tend to improve when a person is calm or focused on an activity.

The types of tics and how often a person has tics changes a lot over time. Even though the symptoms might appear, disappear, and reappear, these conditions are considered chronic.

In most cases, tics decrease during adolescence and early adulthood, and sometimes disappear entirely. However, many people with TS experience tics into adulthood, and in some cases, tics can become worse during adulthood.

Although the media often portray people with TS as involuntarily shouting out swear words (called "coprolalia") or constantly repeating the words of other people (called "echolalia"), these symptoms are rare, and are not required for a diagnosis of TS.

Risk Factors and Causes of Tourette Syndrome

Scientists are studying the causes of and risk factors for TS in an effort to understand it better, and to find better ways to manage TS and to reduce the chances of a person having TS. The causes of TS and other tic disorders are not well-understood.

Although the risk factors for and causes of TS are unknown, current research shows that genes play an important role:

- Genetic studies have indicated that TS is inherited as a dominant gene, with about a 50 percent chance of parents passing the gene on to their children.
- Boys with the gene(s) are three to four times more likely than girls to display symptoms of TS.
- TS can be triggered by abnormal metabolism (breakdown) of a chemical in the brain called "dopamine."

Some research has shown that TS is a genetically complex disorder that likely occurs as a result of the effects of multiple genes interacting with other factors in the environment. Scientists are studying other possible causes and environmental risk factors that might contribute to TS. Some studies have shown that the following factors might be associated with TS, but additional research is needed to better understand these associations:

- Smoking during pregnancy
- Pregnancy complications
- Low birthweight
- Infection. Researchers have found mixed results about whether certain children are more likely to develop tics following infections.

Diagnosis of Tourette Syndrome

There is no single test, like a blood test, to diagnose TS. Health professionals look at the person's symptoms to diagnose TS and other tic disorders. The tic disorders differ from each other in terms of the type of tic present (motor or vocal, or combination of the both), and how long the symptoms have lasted. TS can be diagnosed if a person has both motor and vocal tics, and has had tic symptoms for at least a year.

The American Psychiatric Association's (APA) *Diagnostic and Statistical Manual of Mental Disorders, Fifth Edition* (*DSM-5*) is used by health professionals to help diagnose tic disorders.

Three tic disorders are included in the DSM-5:
- Tourette's disorder (also called "Tourette syndrome")
- Persistent (also called "chronic") motor or vocal tic disorder
- Provisional tic disorder

The tic disorders differ from each other in terms of the type of tic present (motor or vocal, or a combination of both), and how long the symptoms have lasted. People with TS have both motor and vocal tics, and have had tic symptoms for at least 1 year. People with persistent motor or vocal tic disorders have either motor or vocal tics, and have had tic symptoms for at least 1 year. People with provisional tic disorders can have motor or vocal tics, or both, but have had their symptoms less than 1 year.

Here are the criteria in shortened form. Please note that they are presented for your information only and should not be used for self-diagnosis. If you are concerned about any of the symptoms listed, you should consult a trained healthcare provider with experience in diagnosing and treating tic disorders.

Tourette Syndrome

To be diagnosed with TS, a person must:
- Have two or more motor tics (e.g., blinking or shrugging the shoulders) and at least one vocal tic (e.g., humming, clearing the throat, or yelling out a word or phrase), although they might not always happen at the same time
- Have had tics for at least a year. The tics can occur many times a day (usually in bouts) nearly every day, or off and on.
- Have tics that begin before age 18 years
- Have symptoms that are not due to taking medicine or other drugs or due to having another medical condition (e.g., seizures, Huntington disease, or postviral encephalitis)

Persistent (Chronic) Motor or Vocal Tic Disorder

To be diagnosed with a persistent tic disorder, a person must:

- Have one or more motor tics (e.g., blinking or shrugging the shoulders) or vocal tics (e.g., humming, clearing the throat, or yelling out a word or phrase), but not both
- Have tics that occur many times a day nearly every day or on and off throughout a period of more than a year
- Have tics that start before age 18 years
- Have symptoms that are not due to taking medicine or other drugs, or due to having a medical condition that can cause tics (e.g., seizures, Huntington disease, or postviral encephalitis)
- Not have been diagnosed with TS

Provisional Tic Disorder

To be diagnosed with a provisional tic disorder, a person must:

- Have one or more motor tics (e.g., blinking or shrugging the shoulders) or vocal tics (e.g., humming, clearing the throat, or yelling out a word or phrase)
- Have been present for no longer than 12 months in a row
- Have tics that start before age 18 years
- Have symptoms that are not due to taking medicine or other drugs, or due to having a medical condition that can cause tics (e.g., Huntington disease or postviral encephalitis)
- Not have been diagnosed with TS or persistent motor or vocal tic disorder

Treatments of Tourette Syndrome

Although there is no cure for TS, there are treatments to help manage the tics caused by TS. Many people with TS have tics that do not get in the way of their living their daily life and, therefore, do not need any treatment. However, medication and behavioral treatments are available if tics cause pain or injury; interfere with school, work, or social life; or cause stress. A recently developed behavioral treatment is the Comprehensive Behavioral Intervention for Tics (CBIT).

Educating the community (e.g., peers, educators, and coworkers) about TS can increase understanding of the symptoms, reduce teasing, and decrease stress for people living with TS. People with TS cannot help having tics, and are not being disruptive on purpose. When others understand these facts, people with TS might receive more support, which might, in turn, help lessen some tic symptoms.

It is common for people with TS to have co-occurring conditions, particularly attention deficit hyperactivity disorder (ADHD) and obsessive-compulsive disorder (OCD). People with additional conditions will require different treatments based on the symptoms. Sometimes treating these other conditions can help reduce tics. To

As with all medications, those used to treat tics can have side effects. Side effects can include weight gain, stiff muscles, tiredness, restlessness, and social withdrawal. The side effects need to be considered carefully when deciding whether or not to use any medication to treat tics. In some cases, the side effects can be worse than the tics.

Even though medications often are used to treat the symptoms of TS, they might not be helpful for everyone. Two common reasons for not using medications to treat TS are unpleasant side effects and failure of the medications to work as well as expected.

develop the best treatment plan, people with tics, parents, and healthcare providers should work closely with one another, and with everyone involved in treatment and support—which may include teachers, childcare providers, coaches, therapists, and other family members. Taking advantage of all the resources available will help guide success.

Medications

Medications can be used to reduce severe or disruptive tics that might have led to problems in the past with family and friends, other students, or coworkers.

Medications also can be used to reduce symptoms of related conditions, such as ADHD or OCD.

Medications do not eliminate tics completely. However, they can help some people with TS in their everyday life. There is no one medication that is best for all people. Most medications prescribed for TS have not been approved by the U.S. Food and Drug Administration (FDA) for treating tics.

Medications affect each person differently. One person might do well with one medication, but not another. When deciding the best treatment, a doctor might try different medications and doses, and it may take time to find the treatment plan that works best. The doctor will want to find the medication and dose that have the best results and the fewest side effects. Doctors often start with small doses and slowly increase as needed.

Behavioral Therapy

Behavioral therapy is a treatment that teaches people with TS ways to manage their tics. Behavioral therapy is not a cure for tics. However, it can help reduce the number of tics, the severity of tics, the impact of tics, or a combination of all of these. It is important to understand that even though behavioral therapies might help reduce the severity of tics, this does not mean that tics are just psychological or that anyone with tics should be able to control them.

Habit Reversal

Habit reversal is one of the most studied behavioral interventions for people with tics. It has two main parts: awareness training and competing response training. In the awareness training part, people identify each tic out loud. In the competing response part, people learn to do a new behavior that cannot happen at the same time as the tic. For example, if the person with TS has a tic that involves head rubbing, a new behavior might be for that person to place her or his hands on her or his knees, or to cross her or his arms so that the head rubbing cannot take place.

Comprehensive Behavioral Intervention for Tics

Comprehensive Behavioral Intervention for Tics (CBIT) is an evidence-based type of behavioral therapy for TS and chronic tic disorders. CBIT includes habit reversal in addition to other strategies, including education about tics and relaxation techniques. CBIT has been shown to be effective at reducing tic symptoms and tic-related impairment among children and adults.

In CBIT, a therapist will work with a child (and her or his parents) or an adult with TS to better understand the types of tics the person is having and to understand the situations in which the tics are at their worst. Changes to the surroundings may be made, if possible, and the person with TS will also learn to do a new behavior instead of the tic (habit reversal). For example, if a child with TS often has a certain tic during math class, the math teacher can be educated about TS, and perhaps the child's seat can be changed so that the tics are not as visible. In addition, the child also can work with a psychologist to learn habit reversal techniques. This helps to decrease how often the tic occurs by doing a new behavior (like putting her or his hands on her or his knees when an urge to perform the tic happens). CBIT skills can be learned with practice, with the help of an experienced therapist, and with the support and encouragement of those close to the person with TS.

In recent years, more health professionals have recognized that behavioral therapy can be very effective in managing the symptoms of TS. So far, few clinicians have been trained in these types of treatments specifically for TS and tic disorders. The Centers for Disease Control and Prevention (CDC) and The Tourette Association of America have been working to educate more health professionals in this approach to managing TS symptoms.

Parent Training

Children with TS and related conditions and their families also can benefit from parent training, which has been shown to be successful among children with both TS and other disruptive behaviors. Parent training also has been shown to be helpful for children with ADHD. Parent training helps parents better understand their child's behavioral issues and learn parenting skills specific to these problems. The training might include learning about the effective use of positive reinforcement and discipline that is effective with their particular child.

Other Concerns and Conditions

Tourette syndrome often occurs with other related conditions (also called "co-occurring conditions"). These conditions can include ADHD, OCD, and other behavioral or conduct problems. People with TS and related conditions can be at higher risk for learning, behavioral, and social problems.

The symptoms of other disorders can complicate the diagnosis and treatment of TS and create extra challenges for people with TS and their families, educators, and health professionals.

Most children who are diagnosed with TS also have another mental-health, behavioral, or developmental condition.

Conditions that commonly occur with TS include:

- Attention deficit hyperactivity disorder
- Behavioral problems, such as oppositional defiant disorder (ODD) or conduct disorder (CD)
- Anxiety or depression
- Autism spectrum disorder
- Learning disorders
- Speech or language disorders
- Developmental delays or intellectual disabilities

Because co-occurring conditions are so common among people with TS, it is important for doctors to assess every child with TS for other conditions and problems.

Attention Deficit Hyperactivity Disorder

Attention deficit hyperactivity disorder is the most common co-occurring condition among children with TS. Children with ADHD have trouble paying attention and controlling impulsive behaviors. They might act without thinking about what the result will be and, in some cases, they are also overly active. It is normal for children to have trouble focusing and behaving at one time or another. However, for children with ADHD symptoms can continue, can be severe, and cause difficulty at school, at home, or with friends.

Obsessive-Compulsive Behaviors

People with obsessive-compulsive behaviors have unwanted thoughts (obsessions) that they feel a need to respond to (compulsions). Examples of obsessive-compulsive behaviors are having to think about, say, or do something over and over. More than a third of people with TS have OCD. Sometimes it is difficult to tell the difference between complex tics that a child with TS may have and obsessive-compulsive behaviors.

Behavior or Conduct Problems

Oppositional Defiant Disorder

Children with oppositional defiant disorder (ODD) show negative, defiant, and hostile behaviors toward adults or authority figures. ODD usually starts before a child is 8 years of age, but no later than early adolescence. Children with ODD might show symptoms most often with people they know well, such as family members or a regular care provider. The behavior problems associated with ODD are mores severe or persistent than what might be expected for the child's age, and result in major problems in school, at home, or with peers.

Examples of ODD behaviors include:

- Losing one's temper a lot
- Arguing with adults or refusing to comply with adults' rules or requests
- Getting angry or being resentful or vindictive often
- Annoying others on purpose or easily becoming annoyed with others
- Blaming other people often for one's own mistakes or misbehavior

Conduct Disorder

Children with conduct disorder (CD) act aggressive toward others and break rules, laws, and social norms. They might have more injuries and difficulty with friends. In addition, the symptoms of CD happen in more than one area in the child's life (e.g., at home, in the community, and at school).

Behavior problems can be highly disruptive for the child and others in the child's life. It is important to get a diagnosis and treatment plan from a mental-health professional as soon as possible. Effective treatments for disruptive behaviors include behavior therapy training for parents.

Rage

Some people with TS have anger that is out of control, or episodes of "rage." Rage that happens repeatedly and is disproportionate to the situation that triggers it may be diagnosed as a mood disorder, like intermittent explosive disorder. Symptoms might include extreme verbal or physical aggression. Examples of verbal aggression include extreme yelling, screaming, and cursing. Examples of physical aggression include extreme shoving, kicking, hitting, biting, and throwing objects. Rage symptoms are more likely to occur among those with other behavioral disorders such as ADHD, ODD, or CD.

Among people with TS, symptoms of rage are more likely to occur at home than outside the home. Treatment can include behavior therapy, learning how to relax, and social skills training. Some of these methods will help individuals and families better understand what can cause the symptoms of rage, how to avoid encouraging these behaviors, and how to use appropriate discipline for these behaviors. In addition, treating other behavioral disorders that the person might have, such as ADHD, ODD, or CD can help to reduce symptoms of rage.

Anxiety

There are many different types of anxiety disorders with many different causes and symptoms. These include generalized anxiety disorder, OCD, panic disorder, posttraumatic stress disorder, separation anxiety, and different types of phobias. Separation anxiety is most common among young children. These children feel very worried when they are apart from their parents.

Depression

Everyone feels worried, anxious, sad, or stressed from time to time. However, if these feelings do not go away and they interfere with daily life (e.g., keeping a child home from school or other activities, or keeping an adult from working or attending social activities), a person might have depression. Having either a depressed mood or a loss of interest or pleasure for at least 2 weeks might mean that someone has depression. Children and teens with depression might be irritable instead of sad.

To be diagnosed with depression, other symptoms also must be present, such as:
- Changes in eating habits or weight gain or loss
- Changes in sleep habits
- Changes in activity level (others notice increased activity or that the person has slowed down).
- Less energy
- Feelings of worthlessness or guilt
- Difficulty thinking, concentrating, or making decisions
- Repeated thoughts of death
- Thoughts or plans about suicide, or a suicide attempt

Depression can be treated with counseling and medication.

Other Health Concerns

Children with TS can also have other health conditions that require care.

Among the more common health conditions that can occur with TS are:
- Asthma
- Hearing or vision loss
- Bone, joint, or muscle problems
- Brain injury or concussion

A CDC study showed that the rates of asthma and hearing or vision problems were similar to children without TS, but bone, joint, or muscle problems as well as brain injury or concussion were higher for children with TS. Children with TS were also less likely to receive effective coordination of care or have a medical home, which means a primary care setting where a team of providers provides healthcare and preventive services.

Educational Concerns

As a group, people with TS have levels of intelligence similar to those of people without TS. However, people with TS might be more likely to have learning differences, a learning disability, or a developmental delay that affects their ability to learn.

What Is the Best Educational Setting for Children with Tourette Syndrome?

Although students with TS often function well in the regular classroom, ADHD, learning disabilities, obsessive-compulsive symptoms, and frequent tics can greatly interfere with academic performance or social adjustment. After a comprehensive assessment, students should be placed in an educational setting that meets their individual needs. Students may require tutoring, smaller or special classes, and in some cases special schools.

All students with TS need a tolerant and compassionate setting that both encourages them to work to their full potential and is flexible enough to accommodate their special needs. This setting may include a private study area, exams outside the regular classroom, or even oral exams when the child's symptoms interfere with her or his ability to write. Untimed testing reduces stress for students with TS.

(Source: "Tourette Syndrome Fact Sheet," National Institute of Neurological Disorders and Stroke (NINDS))

Many people with TS have problems with writing, organizing, and paying attention. People with TS might have problems processing what they hear or see. This can affect the person's ability to learn by listening to or watching a teacher. Or, the person might have problems with their other senses (such as how things feel, smell, taste, and move) that affects learning and behavior. Children with TS might have trouble with social skills that affect their ability to interact with others.

As a result of these challenges, children with TS might need extra help in school. Many times, these concerns can be addressed with accommodations and behavioral interventions (e.g., help with social skills).

Accommodations can include things such as providing a different testing location or extra testing time, providing tips on how to be more organized, giving the child less homework, or letting the child use a computer to take notes in class. Children also might need behavioral interventions, therapy, or they may need to learn strategies to help with stress, paying attention, or other symptoms.

Who Is Affected?

Studies that included children with diagnosed and undiagnosed TS have estimated that 1 of every 162 children have TS. In the United States, 1 of every 360 children 6 through 17 years of age have been diagnosed with TS, based on parent report. This suggests that about half of children with TS are not diagnosed.

Tourette syndrome can affect people of all racial and ethnic groups. Boys are affected three to five times more often than girls.

CHAPTER 37
LANGUAGE AND SPEECH DISORDERS

It is not unusual for very young children to have difficulty understanding and expressing themselves, but some people continue to experience language problems, often into adolescence and adulthood. Teens with speech and language disorders may have trouble communicating with their peers, teachers, parents, and other adults. As they get older and classroom work requires more advanced oral and written communication skills, their school work may suffer. Beyond that, language disorders in teens can lead to low self-esteem, poor interpersonal relationships, and difficulty in the workforce. When these issues are addressed early through professional intervention, the majority of children show considerable improvement, but for some individuals treatment will continue as they get older, and for those who never received professional attention at a young age, evaluation and treatment may begin during the teen or adult years.

Speech Disorders

A speech disorder is a condition that occurs when a person has difficulty producing the sounds needed to communicate effectively with others. These are often divided into four major types:

- **Articulation.** Articulation refers to the way people make sounds, and those with an articulation disorder may distort, substitute, or leave out some of the sounds used to produce "normal" speech. For example, they may

---

Speech and language disorders are among the most common disabilities facing children and adolescents. According to government statistics, such disorders affect approximately 4.9 percent of U.S. students aged 11 to 17, in addition to even larger numbers of younger children.

(Source: "Quick Statistics about Voice, Speech, Language," National Institute on Deafness and Other Communication Disorders (NIDCD))

substitute a "w" for an "r" ("wobin" for "robin") or leave out a portion of a word ("nana" instead of "banana").

- **Phonology.** Phonological disorders are very closely related to articulation (in fact, many experts classify them together), but phonology refers to the way speech sounds are organized and the way the brain works to sort them out. As children learn to speak, they tend to simplify language in their minds, substituting easier letters for more difficult ones, or just eliminating portions of words to make them easier to say. When individuals do not move beyond this simplification, it is considered a disorder.

- **Voice.** Sometimes called "vocal disorders," these are characterized by the inability to produce a clear sound and can include difficulty with volume, pitch, or other qualities associated with clear communication. Examples include hoarseness, extremely loud speech, very high or low pitch, nasal speech, or occasional total loss of voice.

- **Fluency.** A fluency disorder is one that interferes with the smoothness, continuity, and normal rate of speech. It can include the repetition of sounds or entire words, broken words, gaps in speech, and prolongation of certain sounds. The most common fluency problem is stuttering, which typically begins in childhood and, in some cases, may last a lifetime, to a greater or lesser degree.

Language Disorders

A person with a language disorder has difficulty understanding what is being said by others, finding the right words to communicate clearly, or both. There are three primary types of language disorders:

- **Receptive language disorders.** Individuals with receptive language disorders have problems understanding, retaining, and processing spoken language. Although symptoms vary considerably, they can include appearing not to listen, inability to comprehend complex sentences, difficulty following conversations, and inability to follow instructions.

- **Expressive language disorders.** Those with expressive language disorders have difficulty putting words and sentences together, verbally or in writing, in a cohesive and appropriate manner. The condition is characterized by limited vocabulary, difficulty recalling words, poor grammar, and the inability to put sentences together to tell a coherent story.

- **Mixed receptive-expressive language disorder.** A mixed receptive-expressive language disorder is one in which an individual has trouble both understanding others and expressing herself or himself effectively. The outward characteristics of this condition are essentially the same as those of expressive language disorder, but may also include inappropriate responses to communication or the inability to follow instructions.

Diagnosis

Sometimes speech and language disorders are caused by such conditions as hearing loss, brain injury, neurological problems, or physical issues in the mouth or throat, and in these cases a physician will most likely form a diagnosis. But, more often the cause of the disorder is unknown, making diagnosis by a trained specialist necessary.

There are a number of standardized tests specifically aimed at children from birth to six years of age that are routinely administered to arrive at a diagnosis and help develop a treatment plan. Even though there has been less attention paid to the formal evaluation of speech and language issues in teens, there are some standardized tests that, combined with general observation, interviews, and a review of classroom performance, can be useful in obtaining a diagnosis. Some of these include:

- **Peabody Picture Test.** Designed in 1959 and updated several times since then, this test is administered to children, teens, and adults to determine receptive vocabulary ability. During the test, the examiner shows the individual being evaluated a series of pictures then says a word and has the subject identify the picture that best illustrates the word. Results are then compared to standardized norms for the age group.
- **The Listening Comprehension Test Adolescent.** Intended for individuals aged 12 to 17, this test evaluates the student's ability to listen and comprehend language that would typically be used in a classroom setting. During testing, the subject listens to a story and then answers questions posed by the examiner, some of which relate to understanding of the story's meaning, some to vocabulary, and others to recall information.
- **The Word Test 2 Adolescent.** This test measures an individual's ability to understand the meaning of words, using six skill areas to evaluate both classroom and common language usage. These include identifying a synonym for a given word, providing an antonym for a given word, choosing the unrelated word among four, defining words, repairing an absurd statement, and giving multiple meanings for words.
- **Social Language Development Test Adolescent.** This evaluation assesses such areas as the teen's ability to interpret social language, engage in social interactions, take on someone else's perspective, and devise solutions to social problems based on language used in the interaction. The procedure involves a variety of pictures, stories, and role-playing exercises.

There are many other tests that professionals who specialize in working with teens may use to help diagnose speech and language problems, including those that evaluate spelling, writing, reading comprehension, memory, and vocabulary.

Public schools can help teens with speech and language disorders in a number of ways. Qualified students can work with their parents, educators, and professionals to develop an Individualized Education Program (IEP), which could include classroom assistance, homework plans, and speech therapy.

Treatment

Because of the complexity and numerous types of speech and language disorders, treatment plans vary considerably from case to case. Ideally, the cooperation of specialized professionals, parents, school systems, teachers, and peers will help ensure the best possible outcome:

- Speech therapists and language specialists can work individually with the student to help improve pronunciation, vocabulary, and grammar skills.
- Psychologists may be engaged if the student has emotional issues related to, or underlying, speech or language disorders.
- Public schools are required under the Individuals with Disabilities Education Act (IDEA) to provide special educational programs (SEPs) for qualified individuals, so those with language disorders might be able to get help through the school system.
- Although teachers may not be specially trained in speech therapy, after discussions with parents and professionals, they will likely be able to make accommodations for students who have language difficulty. For example, they might allow alternative means of communication for some students, or they could modify homework assignments to meet those students' needs.
- Peers can be a great source of practice or reinforcement. Those who have speech or language disorders themselves can form part of a network to work with each other on various exercises. And peers who do not have such disorders can be enlisted to serve as role models and sources of feedback for their friends or classmates who need extra help in this area.

References

1. Clark, Mary Kristen, MS; Alan G. Kamhi, Ph.D. "Language Disorders," International Encyclopedia of Rehabilitation, 2010.
2. Elleseff, Tatyana, MA, CCC-SLP. "Comprehensive Assessment of Adolescents with Suspected Language and Literacy Disorders," SmartSpeechTherapy.com, October 9, 2016.
3. "Speech and Language Disorders," Bright Minds Institute, n.d.
4. "Speech and Language Impairments," Center for Parent Information and Resources (CPIR), January 2011.
5. "Speech and Language Therapy," Kaufman Children's Center (KCC), 2016.
6. "Understanding Language Disorders," Understood.org, n.d.

CHAPTER 38
HEARING LOSS

About This Chapter: This chapter includes text excerpted from "Hearing Loss in Children—What Is Hearing Loss in Children?" Centers for Disease Control and Prevention (CDC), June 8, 2020.

Hearing Loss in Children

Hearing loss can affect a child's ability to develop speech, language, and social skills. The earlier children with hearing loss start getting services, the more likely they are to reach their full potential. If you think that a child might have hearing loss, ask the child's doctor for a hearing screening as soon as possible. Do not wait!

What Is Hearing Loss?

A hearing loss can happen when any part of the ear is not working in the usual way. This includes the outer ear, middle ear, inner ear, hearing (acoustic) nerve, and auditory system.

Signs and Symptoms of Hearing Loss

The signs and symptoms of hearing loss are different for each child. If you think that your child might have hearing loss, ask the child's doctor for a hearing screening as soon as possible. Do not wait!

Even if a child has passed a hearing screening before, it is important to look out for the following signs.

Signs in Babies

- Does not startle at loud noises
- Does not turn to the source of a sound after 6 months of age
- Does not say single words, such as "dada" or "mama" by 1 year of age
- Turns head when she or he sees you but not if you only call out her or his name. This sometimes is mistaken for not paying attention or just ignoring, but could be the result of a partial or complete hearing loss.
- Seems to hear some sounds but not others

Signs in Children

- Speech is delayed
- Speech is not clear
- Does not follow directions. This sometimes is mistaken for not paying attention or just ignoring, but could be the result of a partial or complete hearing loss.
- Often says, "Huh?"
- Turns the TV volume up too high

Babies and children should reach milestones in how they play, learn, communicate, and act. A delay in any of these milestones could be a sign of hearing loss or other developmental problem.

Screening and Diagnosis of Hearing Loss

Hearing Screening

Hearing screening is a test to tell if people might have hearing loss. Hearing screening is easy and not painful. In fact, babies are often asleep while being screened. It takes a very short time—usually only a few minutes.

Babies

- All babies should be screened for hearing loss no later than 1 month of age. It is best if they are screened before leaving the hospital after birth.
- If a baby does not pass a hearing screening, it is very important to get a full hearing test as soon as possible, but no later than 3 months of age.

Older Babies and Children

- If you think a child might have hearing loss, ask the doctor for a hearing test as soon as possible.
- Children who are at risk for acquired, progressive, or delayed-onset hearing loss should have at least one hearing test by 2 to 2 1/2 years of age. Hearing loss that gets worse over time is known as "acquired or progressive hearing loss." Hearing loss that develops after the baby is born is called "delayed-onset hearing loss."
- If a child does not pass a hearing screening, it is very important to get a full hearing test as soon as possible.

Full Hearing Test

All children who do not pass a hearing screening should have a full hearing test. This test is also called an "audiology evaluation." An audiologist, who is an expert trained to test hearing, will do the full hearing test. In addition, the audiologist will also ask questions about birth history, ear infection, and hearing loss in the family.

There are many kinds of tests an audiologist can do to find out if a person has a hearing loss, how much of a hearing loss there is, and what type it is. The hearing tests are easy and not painful.

Some of the tests the audiologist might use include:

Auditory Brainstem Response Test or Brainstem Auditory Evoked Response Test

- Auditory brainstem response (ABR) or brainstem auditory evoked response (BAER) is a test that checks the brain's response to sound. Because this test does not rely on a person's response behavior, the person being tested can be sound asleep during the test.

Otoacoustic Emissions

Otoacoustic emissions (OAE) is a test that checks the inner ear response to sound. Because this test does not rely on a person's response behavior, the person being tested can be sound asleep during the test.

Behavioral Audiometry Evaluation

Behavioral audiometry evaluation will test how a person responds to sound overall. Behavioral audiometry evaluation tests the function of all parts of the ear. The person being tested must be awake and actively respond to sounds heard during the test.

With the parents' permission, the audiologist will share the results with the child's primary care doctor and other experts, such as:

- An ear, nose, and throat doctor, also called an "otolaryngologist"
- An eye doctor, also called an "ophthalmologist"
- A professional trained in genetics, also called a "clinical geneticist" or a "genetics counselor"

Treatment and Intervention Services of Hearing Loss

No single treatment or intervention is the answer for every child or family. Good intervention plans will include close monitoring, follow-ups and any changes needed along the way. There are many different options for children with hearing loss and their families.

Some of the treatment and intervention options include:

- Working with a professional (or team) who can help a child and family learn to communicate
- Getting a hearing device, such as a hearing aid
- Joining support groups
- Taking advantage of other resources available to children with a hearing loss and their families

Early Intervention and Special Education

Early Intervention (0 to 3 Years)

Hearing loss can affect a child's ability to develop speech, language, and social skills. The earlier a child who is deaf or hard of hearing starts getting services, the more likely the child's speech, language, and social skills will reach their full potential.

Early intervention program services help young children with hearing loss learn language skills and other important skills. Research shows that early intervention services can greatly improve a child's development.

Babies who are diagnosed with hearing loss should begin to get intervention services as soon as possible, but no later than 6 months of age.

There are many services available through the Individuals with Disabilities Education Improvement Act 2004 (IDEA 2004) (sites.ed.gov/idea). Services for children from birth through 36 months of age are called "early intervention" or "Part C" services. Even if your child has not been diagnosed with a hearing loss, she or he may be eligible for early intervention treatment services. The IDEA 2004 says that children under the age of 3 years (36 months) who are at risk of having developmental delays may be eligible for services. These services are provided through an early intervention system in your state. Through this system, you can ask for an evaluation.

Special Education (3 to 22 Years)

Special education is instruction specifically designed to address the educational and related developmental needs of older children with disabilities, or those who are experiencing developmental delays. Services for these children are provided through the public school system. These services are available through the Individuals with Disabilities Education Improvement Act 2004 (IDEA 2004), Part B.

Early Hearing Detection and Intervention Program

Every state has an Early Hearing Detection and Intervention (EHDI) program. EHDI works to identify infants and children with hearing loss. EHDI also promotes timely follow-up testing and services or interventions for any family whose child has a hearing loss. If your child has a hearing loss or if you have any concerns about your child's hearing, call toll-free at 800-CDC-INFO (800-232-4636) or contact your local EHDI program coordinator (www.infanthearing.org/status/cnhs.php) to find available services in your state.

Technology

Many people who are deaf or hard of hearing have some hearing. The amount of hearing a deaf or hard of hearing person has is called "residual hearing."

Technology does not "cure" hearing loss, but may help a child with hearing loss to make the most of their residual hearing. For those parents who choose to have their child use technology, there are many options, including:

- Hearing aids

- Cochlear or brainstem implants
- Bone-anchored hearing aids
- Other assistive devices

Hearing Aids

Hearing aids make sounds louder. They can be worn by people of any age, including infants. Babies with hearing loss may understand sounds better using hearing aids. This may give them the chance to learn speech skills at a young age.

There are many styles of hearing aids. They can help many types of hearing losses. A young child is usually fitted with behind-the-ear style hearing aids because they are better suited to growing ears.

Cochlear and Auditory Brainstem Implants

A cochlear implant may help many children with severe to profound hearing loss—even very young children. It gives that child a way to hear when a hearing aid is not enough. Unlike a hearing aid, cochlear implants do not make sounds louder. A cochlear implant sends sound signals directly to the hearing nerve.

Persons with severe to profound hearing loss due to an absent or very small hearing nerve or severely abnormal inner ear (cochlea), may not benefit from a hearing aid or cochlear implant. Instead, an auditory brainstem implant may provide some hearing. An auditory brainstem implant directly stimulates the hearing pathways in the brainstem, bypassing the inner ear and hearing nerve.

Both cochlear and brainstem implants have two main parts—the parts that are placed inside the inner ear, the cochlea, or base of the brain, the brainstem ear during surgery, and the parts that are worn outside the ear after surgery. The parts outside the ear send sounds to the parts inside the ear.

Bone-Anchored Hearing Aids

This type of hearing aid can be considered when a child has either a conductive, mixed or unilateral hearing loss and is specifically suitable for children who cannot otherwise wear 'in the ear' or 'behind the ear' hearing aids.

Other Assistive Devices

Besides hearing aids, there are other devices that help people with hearing loss. Following are some examples of other assistive devices:

Frequency Modulation System

Frequency modulation (FM) system is a kind of device that helps people with hearing loss hear in background noise. FM stands for "frequency modulation." It is the same type of signal used for radios. FM systems send sound from a microphone used by someone speaking to a person wearing the receiver. This system is sometimes used with hearing aids. An extra piece is attached to the hearing aid that works with the FM system.

Captioning

Many television programs, videos, and DVDs are captioned. Television sets made after 1993 are made to show the captioning. You do not have to buy anything special. Captions show the conversation spoken in soundtrack of a program on the bottom of the television screen.

Other Devices

There are many other devices available for children with hearing loss. Some of these include:

- Text messaging
- Telephone amplifiers
- Flashing and vibrating alarms
- Audio loop systems
- Infrared listening devices
- Portable sound amplifiers
- TTY (Text telephone or teletypewriter)

Medical and Surgical

Medications or surgery may also help make the most of a person's hearing. This is especially true for a conductive hearing loss, or one that involves a part of the outer or middle ear that is not working in the usual way.

One type of conductive hearing loss can be caused by a chronic ear infection. A chronic ear infection is a build-up of fluid behind the eardrum in the middle ear space. Most ear infections are managed with medication or careful monitoring. Infections that do not go away with medication can be treated with a simple surgery that involves putting a tiny tube into the eardrum to drain the fluid out.

Another type of conductive hearing loss is caused by either the outer and/or middle ear not forming correctly while the baby was growing in the mother's womb. Both the outer and middle ear need to work together in order for sound to be sent correctly to the inner ear. If any of these parts did not form correctly, there might be a hearing loss in that ear. This problem may be improved and perhaps even corrected with surgery. An ear, nose, and throat doctor (otolaryngologist) is the healthcare professional who usually takes care of this problem.

Placing a cochlear implant, auditory brainstem implant, or bone-anchored hearing aid will also require a surgery.

Learning Language

Without extra help, children with hearing loss have problems learning language. These children can then be at risk for other delays. Families who have children with hearing loss often need to change their communication habits or learn special skills (such as sign language) to help their children learn language. These skills can be used together with hearing aids, cochlear or auditory brainstem implants, and other devices that help children hear.

Family Support Services

For many parents, their child's hearing loss is unexpected. Parents sometimes need time and support to adapt to the child's hearing loss.

Parents of children with recently identified hearing loss can seek different kinds of support. Support is anything that helps a family and may include advice, information, having the chance to get to know other parents who have a child with hearing loss, locating a deaf mentor, finding childcare or transportation, giving parents time for personal relaxation, or just a supportive listener.

How People with Hearing Loss Learn Language

People with hearing loss and their families often need special skills to be able to learn language and communicate. These skills can be used together with hearing aids, cochlear implants, and other devices that help people hear. There are several approaches that can help, each emphasizing different language learning skills.

Some families choose a single approach because that is what works best for them. Other people choose skills from two or more approaches because that is what works best for them.

Following are language approaches, and the skills that are sometimes included in each of them:

- **Auditory-oral**
  - Natural gestures, listening, speech (lip) reading, spoken speech
- **Auditory-verbal**
  - Listening, spoken speech
- **Bilingual**
  - American sign language (ASL) and English
- **Cued speech**
  - Cueing, speech (lip) reading
- **Total communication**
  - Conceptually Accurate Signed English (CASE), Signing Exact English (SEE), finger spelling, listening, Manually Coded English (MCE), natural gestures, speech (lip) reading, spoken speech

Communication Tools

American Sign Language

American sign language is a language itself. While English and Spanish are spoken languages, ASL is a visual language.

American sign language is a complete language. People communicate using hand shapes, direction and motion of the hands, body language, and facial expressions. ASL has its own grammar, word order, and sentence structure. People can share feelings, jokes, and complete ideas using ASL.

Like any other language, ASL must be learned. People can take ASL classes and start teaching their baby even while they are still learning it. A baby can learn ASL as a first language. Also, experts in ASL can work with families to help them learn ASL.

Children can use many other skills with ASL. Finger spelling is one skill that is almost always used with ASL. Finger spelling is used to spell out words that do not have a sign—such as names of people and places.

Manually Coded English

Manually Coded English (MCE) is made up of signs that are a visual code for spoken English. MCE is a code for a language—the English language. Many of the signs (hand shapes and hand motions) in MCE are borrowed from ASL. But unlike ASL, the grammar, word order, and sentence structure of MCE are similar to the English language.

Children and adults can use many other communication tools along with MCE. One that is commonly used is finger spelling, which is used to spell out words that do not have a sign in MCE—such as names of people and places.

Conceptually Accurate Signed English

Conceptually Accurate Signed English (CASE) (sometimes called "Pidgin Signed English" (PSE)) has developed between people who use ASL, and people who use Manually Coded English (MCE), using signs based on ASL and MCE. This helps them understand each other better. CASE is flexible, and can be changed depending on the people using it.

Other communication tools can be used with CASE. Often, finger spelling is used in combination with CASE. Finger spelling is used to spell out words that do not have a sign, such as names of people and places.

Cued Speech

Cued speech helps people who are deaf or hard of hearing better understand spoken languages.

When watching a person's mouth, many speech sounds look the same on the face even though the sounds heard are not the same. For instance, the words "mat," "bat," and "pat," look the same on the face even though they sound very different. When "cueing" English, the person communicating uses eight hand shapes and four places near the mouth to help the person looking tell the difference between speech sounds. Cued speech allows the person to make out sounds and words when they are using other building blocks, such as speech reading (lip reading) or auditory training (listening).

Finger Spelling

With finger spelling the person uses hands and fingers to spell out words. Hand shapes represent the letters in the alphabet. Finger spelling is used with many other communication methods; it is almost never used by itself. It is most often used with ASL, Conceptually Accurate Signed English (CASE), and Manually Coded English (MCE) to spell out words that do not have a sign, such as the names of places or people.

Natural Gestures

"Natural gestures"—or body language—are actions that people normally do to help others understand a message. For example, if a parent wants to ask a toddler if she or he wants to be picked up, the parent might stretch out her or his arms and ask, "Up?" For an older child, the parent might motion with her or his arms as she or he calls the child to come inside. Or, the parent might put a first finger over her or his mouth and nose to show that the child needs to be quiet.

Babies will begin to use this building block naturally if they can see what others are doing. This building block is not taught, it just comes naturally. It is always used with other building blocks.

Listening/Auditory Training

Most people who are deaf or hard of hearing have some hearing. This is called "residual hearing." Some people rely or learn how to maximize their residual hearing (auditory training). This building block is often used in combination with other building blocks (such as hearing aids, cochlear implants, and other assistive devices).

Listening might seem easy to a person with hearing. But for a person with hearing loss, listening is often hard without proper training. Like all other tools, the skill of listening must be learned. Often a speech-language pathologist (a professional trained to teach people how to use speech and language) will work with the person with hearing loss and the family.

Spoken Speech

People can use speech to express themselves. Speech is a skill that many people take for granted. Learning to speak is a skill that can help build language.

Speech or learning to speak is often used in combination with hearing aids, cochlear implants, and other assistive devices that help people maximize their residual hearing. A person with some residual hearing may find it easier to learn speech than a person with no residual hearing. Since speech can only be used by a person to express herself or himself other building blocks, such as hearing with a hearing aid, must be added in order to help the person understands what is being said so they can communicate with others.

Speaking may seem easy to a person with hearing. But for a person with hearing loss, speaking is often hard without proper training. Like all other communication tools, the skill of speaking must be learned. Often a speech-language pathologist (a professional trained to teach people how to use speech and language) will work with the person with hearing loss and the family.

Speech Reading

Speech reading (or lip reading) helps a person with hearing loss understand speech. The person watches the movements of a speaker's mouth and face, and understands what the speaker is saying. About 40 percent of the sounds in the English language can be seen on the lips of a speaker in good conditions, such as a well-lit room where the child can see the speaker's face. But some words cannot be read. For example: "bop," "mop," and "pop," look exactly alike when spoken. (You can see this for yourself in a mirror). A good speech reader might be able to see only 4 to 5 words in a 12-word sentence.

Children often use speech reading in combination with other tools, such as auditory training (listening), cued speech, and others. But it cannot be successful alone. Babies will naturally begin using this building block if they can see the speaker's mouth and face. But as a child gets older, she or he will still need some training.

Sometimes, when talking with a person who is deaf or hard of hearing, people will exaggerate their mouth movements or talk very loudly. Exaggerated mouth movements and a loud voice can make speech reading very hard. It is important to talk in a normal way and look directly at your child's face and make sure she or he is watching you.

Causes and Risk Factors of Hearing Loss

Hearing loss can happen any time during life—from before birth to adulthood.

Following are some of the things that can increase the chance that a child will have hearing loss:

- **A genetic cause.** About 1 out of 2 cases of hearing loss in babies is due to genetic causes. Some babies with a genetic cause for their hearing loss might have family members who also have a hearing loss. About 1 out of 3 babies with genetic hearing loss have a "syndrome." This means they have other conditions in addition to the hearing loss, such as Down syndrome or Usher syndrome.
- 1 out of 4 cases of hearing loss in babies is due to maternal infections during pregnancy, complications after birth, and head trauma. For example, the child:
  - Was exposed to infection, such as, before birth
  - Spent 5 days or more in a hospital neonatal intensive care unit (NICU) or had complications while in the NICU
  - Needed a special procedure like a blood transfusion to treat bad jaundice
  - Has head, face, or ears shaped or formed in a different way than usual
  - Has a condition like a neurological disorder that may be associated with hearing loss
  - Had an infection around the brain and spinal cord called "meningitis"
  - Received a bad injury to the head that required a hospital stay
- For about 1 out of 4 babies born with hearing loss, the cause is unknown.

Prevention of Hearing Loss

Following are tips for parents to help prevent hearing loss in their children:

Get Help!
- If you think that your child might have hearing loss, ask the child's doctor for a **hearing screening** as soon as possible. Do not wait!
- If your child does not pass a hearing screening, ask the child's doctor for a **full hearing test** as soon as possible.
- If your child has hearing loss, talk to the child's doctor about **treatment and intervention services**.

- Have a healthy pregnancy.
- Make sure your child gets all the regular childhood vaccines.
- Keep your child away from high noise levels, such as from very loud toys.

CHAPTER 39
PEDIATRIC SLEEP-DISORDERED BREATHING

Breathing trouble that is experienced by children during sleep is termed as "pediatric sleep-disordered breathing" (SDB). It can involve loud snoring as well as obstructive sleep apnea (OSA), which is a condition where the airway is repeatedly blocked during sleep. About 10 percent of children snore daily, and around 2 to 4 percent of children suffer from OSA. It also causes behavioral changes during the day such as lethargy or hyperactivity. During such times, the child experiences increased heart rate and blood pressure. Additionally, the brain is aroused, sleep is disrupted, and in some cases, the oxygen level in the blood is considerably reduced.

Symptoms of Pediatric Sleep-Disordered Breathing
Pediatric SDB has a severe impact on children that influences their performance in every aspect of development and education. This can lead to an adverse effect on the health of the child well into adulthood. The following are the potential symptoms of pediatric SDB:

1. **Snoring.** It is the most common symptom of SDB that affects a child during most of the nights. Loud snoring can often be interrupted by a complete obstruction of breathing, involving gasping and snorting as well as waking up from sleep.

2. **Irritability.** Children with SDB often become irritable, have trouble focusing at school, have increased day time fatigue, and exhibit hyperactive behavior.

3. **Enuresis.** Also known as "bed-wetting," occurs due to increased urine production during the night.

4. **Learning trouble.** SDB causes kids to become disruptive and moody at home and school, which results in attention deficit disorders in some children.
5. **Slow development.** Children produce fewer growth hormones and this results in unusually slow development and growth.
6. **Cardiovascular problems.** An increased risk of high blood pressure or other heart and lung problems that occur due to OSA.

Causes of Pediatric Sleep-Disordered Breathing

Sleep-disordered breathing is most commonly caused by the narrowing of airways due to enlarged tonsils and adenoids, which is a patch of tissue behind the nasal cavity. Children who are obese are at most risk for SDB as a result of fat deposits around the throat and neck. A few other risk factors of pediatric SDB include:

- Down syndrome
- Skull or face abnormalities
- Sickle cell disease
- Neuromuscular disorders such as cerebral palsy
- Low birth weight
- Family history of OSA

Treatment of Pediatric Sleep-Disordered Breathing

The enlarged tonsils and adenoids, which cause SDB, can be surgically removed using a procedure known as "tonsillectomy and adenoidectomy" (T&A). Long-term improvement can be seen in most children's sleep and behavior after performing the T&A procedure. However, if the symptoms are not severe, the tonsils are small or the child is nearing puberty and both tonsils and adenoids shrink during puberty and require no surgery. Mild symptoms do not affect the academic performance and behavior of the child; however, they should be constantly observed to ensure the symptoms do not worsen. In some cases, further treatments including weight loss, additional surgical procedures, and the usage of continuous positive airway pressure (CPAP) is found to be beneficial.

References

1. "Pediatric Sleep-Disordered Breathing," American Academy of Otolaryngology-Head and Neck Surgery Foundation (AAO-HNSF), October 4, 2018.
2. "Pediatric Obstructive Sleep Apnea," Mayo Foundation for Medical Education and Research (MFMER), September 18, 2018.
3. "Pediatric Sleep-Disordered Breathing/Obstructive Sleep Apnea," Boston Medical Center (BMC), November 16, 2011.

PART 5 | SCHOOL OPTIONS FOR TEENS WITH LEARNING DISABILITY

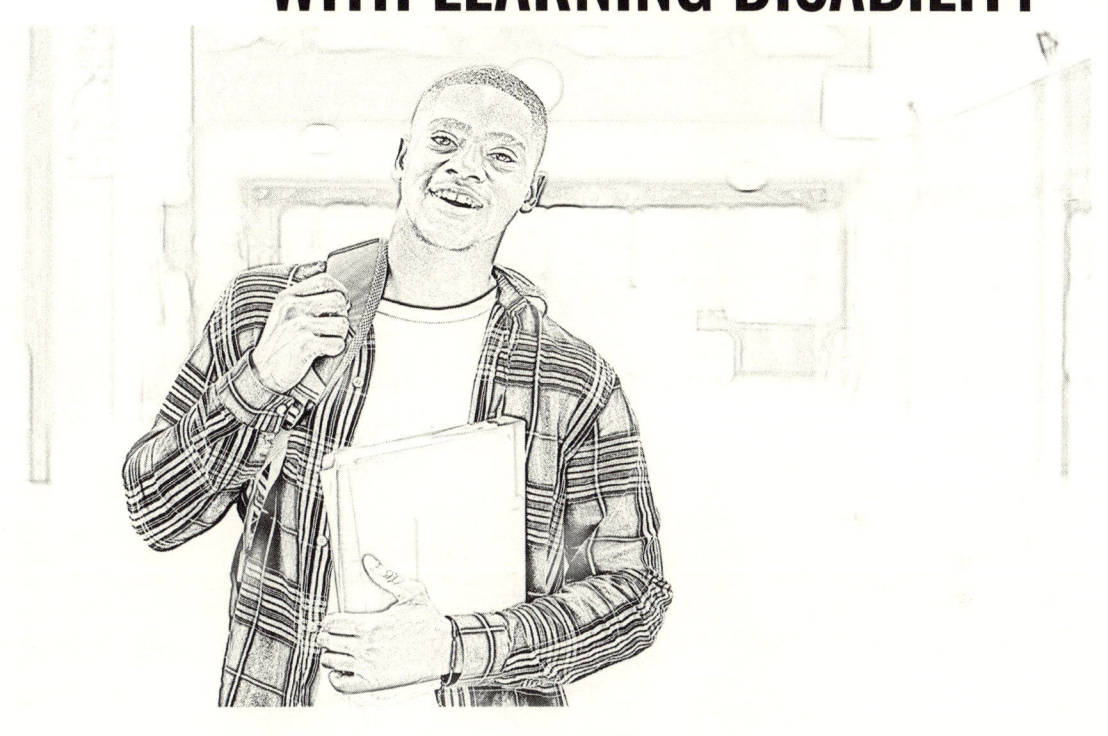

CHAPTER 40
CHOOSING A SCHOOL

About This Chapter: "Choosing a School," © 2017 Omnigraphics. Reviewed July 2020.

Today there is a dizzying array of options available when it comes to choosing a school for students with learning disabilities (LDs). These range from regular classrooms with trained staff support to ordinary schools with dedicated special-needs programs to specialized schools for students with LD. Although this is certainly a good thing, it also creates a daunting task for parents and teens attempting to sort through the choices.

The first step is to have the student's LD properly assessed, if this has not already been done. An accurate evaluation is necessary in order to focus on those schools or programs that are best suited to the student's particular needs. Testing can be done through public programs or privately by a licensed professional—usually a clinical psychologist, an educational psychologist, or a neuropsychologist—and generally consists of evaluating overall intelligence, memory, reasoning, achievement and ability in various areas, verbal skills, and physical ability.

Types of Schools for Students with Learning Disability

Once the assessment process is complete, the professionals who analyzed the results will go over their findings and can help with recommendations for the type of school that is most appropriate for the student. These may include:

Before the passage of The Individuals with Disabilities Education Act (formerly called the "Education for All Handicapped Children Act"), just one in five students with physical, psychological, or learning disabilities were being educated in U.S. schools. This legislation requires that all students receive free access to an appropriate education.
(Source: "Archived: A 25 Year History of the IDEA," U.S. Department of Education (ED))

- **Public schools.** Neighborhood schools have several immediate advantages: they are close to home, are free, and allow the teen to interact with many different types of students. They are also required by law to give the student an appropriate education, which means helping develop an appropriate program to meet her or his needs. This can include special support in a regular classroom, dedicated classes for students with similar needs, and specially trained staff. But, public schools can vary considerably in available resources for students with LD, and possible downsides include less individual attention due to large class sizes and few special-education teachers on staff.

- **Charter schools and magnet schools.** These still operate under the public-school system, which means there is no charge to attend. Some focus on specific areas of education, so it is possible to select one that aligns with the student's academic strengths, yet they also provide support for those with learning disabilities. In addition, the class sizes tend to be smaller, and some of these schools even focus specifically on students with LD. On the other hand, they may not be near the student's home, can have waiting lists for admission, and, in the case of charter schools, which are run by private or community groups, might have limited funding available for LD education.

- **Private schools.** Private schools almost always have smaller class sizes, which allows for more individual attention. They can also provide a different type of education than is found in public schools, such as religious instruction or a focus on specific subjects. And although private schools are not required by law to provide services to students with LD, some may be equipped to do so, and in other cases, the student might be eligible to receive these services through the local public school. Of course, private schools charge tuition, which may be very expensive, although scholarships and financial aid could be available.

- **Private schools for students with LD.** Most students with LD attend ordinary schools, but some want or need a school that specializes in teaching students with their disability. These schools are able to provide the most support, with teachers and staff who have the most comprehensive training, as well as curricula and programs that have been specifically designed for students with LD. In addition, the environment is generally more welcoming to individuals with disabilities, and other students tend to be more accepting of their peers. However, in this type of school, the student's interaction will be limited to others with learning disabilities, which can be a drawback to social development. And, again, tuition can be expensive, but in some cases, the local school system might assume the expense if it is not able to provide an appropriate education elsewhere.

The field of special education is constantly evolving, so schools need to ensure that teachers are up-to-date on the latest research and methods. Before deciding on a school, ask about its program for the ongoing development of staff.

- **Homeschooling.** Although it is not for everyone, homeschooling can provide certain advantages for both parents and students. For example, individual attention is maximized, coursework can be tailored to the student's needs, and some issues, like bullying, can be eliminated. Of course homeschooling requires an intense commitment—in both time and energy—on the part of the parent or other person who will be responsible for the LD student's education. There is also the need to ensure that the student interacts regularly with other individuals, her or his own age through outside activities.

Steps in Choosing a School

Once the type of school has been determined, based on the particular needs and preferences of the LD student and parents, the next task is to decide on a specific school. Some steps include:

- **Gather information.** The phone book might be one place to start. But, a more focused plan might be to ask for recommendations from the health or educational professional who currently works with the LD student, from another parent or student, or from the local chapter of the Learning Disabilities Association of America.
- **Narrow down the choices.** This is a good time to use the Internet or consult published sources for pluses and minuses about the various schools under consideration. It is also a good idea to collect pamphlets or other written information from various schools, check school ratings and evaluations, and even attend parent fairs and open houses. If possible, talk to parents and students who are familiar with these schools for personal opinions.
- **Investigate the school.** Once a potential choice has been identified, it is time to burrow down into the details. Find out if the school is properly accredited, read the school's mission statement (usually available on its website), explore teacher requirements and certifications, learn about special programs and extracurricular activities that might benefit the student. And, finally, visit the school, ideally more than once. Observe a typical day, get a feel of the environment, check out the classrooms and see what technology is in use there, and, if possible, sit in on a class or two. Meet with the head of the school, some of the teachers, and, if this can be arranged, a current student and his or her parents. Ask as many

questions as possible about the curriculum, teaching methods, programs and facilities devoted to the student's particular LD, the school's daily routine, how behavioural issues are handled, communication style, family involvement, and any other areas of concern.

References

1. Blake, Hannah. "Choosing the Right School for Your Child with Learning Difficulties or a Learning Disability," MadeForMums.com, n.d.
2. Chaban, Peter. "Choosing the Right School for Special Needs Children," AboutKidsHealth.ca, September 3, 2010.
3. Dwight, Valle. "Special Needs Programs and Schools: A Primer," GreatSchools org, April 30, 2015.
4. Tucker, Geri Coleman. "Choosing a School: Know the Options for Your Child," Understood.org, March 30, 2014.
5. Weston, Susan Perkins; Joe Nathan; Mary Anne Raywid. "Choosing a School for Your Child," Office of Educational Research and Improvement (OERI), U.S. Department of Education (ED), 2005.

CHAPTER 41
SPECIAL EDUCATION SERVICES

About This Chapter: This chapter includes text excerpted from "Youth with Disabilities—Introduction," Youth.gov, October 3, 2012. Reviewed July 2020.

Special Education Services for Children and Youth

Youth who receive special education services under the Individuals with Disabilities Education Act (IDEA 2004), and especially young adults of transition age, should be involved in planning for life after high school as early as possible and no later than age 16. Young adults of transition age who have disabilities should not only be invited to attend their Individualized Education Plan (IEP) meetings, but be supported as key decision-makers in order to ensure their plans for high school and life after high school are based on their interests and strengths.

The IDEA 2004 includes requirements for special education and related services for children and youth. The federal language uses the term "child" to mean individuals ages 3 to 21 and provides the following clarifying definition of whom the law applies:

- Child with a disability means a child evaluated in accordance with Sec. 300.304 through 300.311 as having mental retardation, a hearing impairment (including deafness), a speech or language impairment, a visual impairment (including blindness), a serious emotional disturbance (referred to in this part as "emotional disturbance"), an orthopedic impairment, autism, traumatic brain injury (TBI), other health impairment, a specific learning disability, deaf-blindness, or multiple disabilities, and who, by reason thereof, needs special education and related services.

Transition Age Youth with Disabilities

Transition age youth with disabilities receive a continuum of supports and services designed to address their specific needs, interests, strengths, and educational goals. Teachers, service providers, clinicians, family members, and the student herself or himself work together to develop a coordinated plan for service delivery and strategize about how best to meet the student's social, emotional, physical, and educational needs. Approximately six percent of children and youth ages 5 to 20 live with some type of disability. While their needs and postsecondary goals may vary, each young person needs individualized support and guidance in planning for life beyond high school.

Recognizing the importance of maintaining a continuum of services beyond high school and into adulthood, federal disability legislation requires the inclusion of transition planning in each child's IEP. By the time a student reaches the age of 16 (if not before), the IEP must include measurable postsecondary goals and identify appropriate transition services. According to the accompanying regulations for IDEA 2004, "transition services" means a coordinated set of activities for a child with a disability that:

- Is designed to be within a results-oriented process that is focused on improving the academic and functional achievement of the child with a disability to facilitate the child's movement from school to postschool activities, including postsecondary education, vocational education, integrated employment (including supported employment), continuing and adult education, adult services, independent living, and community participation;
- Is based on the individual child's needs, taking into account the child's strengths, preferences, and interests; and
- Includes instruction, related services, community experiences, the development of employment and other postschool adult living objectives, and, if appropriate, acquisition of daily living skills and functional vocational evaluation.

Transition services should stem from the individual youth's needs and strengths, ensuring that planning takes into account her or his interests, preferences, and desires for the future.

CHAPTER 42
SCHOOL-BASED PREPARATORY EXPERIENCES

About This Chapter: This chapter includes text excerpted from "Youth in Transition," U.S. Department of Labor (DOL), July 25, 2019.

In order to perform at optimal levels in all education settings, all youth need to participate in educational programs grounded in standards, clear performance expectations, and graduation exit options based upon meaningful, accurate, and relevant indicators of student learning and skills. These should include:

- Ability to perform academically at or above proficiency for grade level
- Ability to perform academically at levels equivalent to college readiness standards by the time of high school completion (e.g., requiring no remediation upon postsecondary enrollment)
- Motivation and persistence toward academic goals
- Knowledge about education and career options and ability to make informed decisions about academic courses and postsecondary plans to achieve individualized academic, career, and life goals
- Ability to manage academic and nonacademic challenges that impede learning using competencies such as social and emotional learning skills, self-direction and learning habits, self-determination, and self-advocacy
- Social and emotional skills including self-awareness, self-management, social awareness, relationship skills, problem-solving, conflict resolution, and responsible decision-making
- Skills and knowledge needed to effectively use technology for a variety of purposes, including test-taking, online classes, organization, time management, or performing tasks in one's field of study or career path
- Ability to advocate for oneself in secondary and postsecondary planning processes and learning environments

High School/High Tech

The High School/High Tech (HS/HT) program provides opportunities for students with all types of disabilities to explore exciting careers in science, mathematics, and technology. The program is one of several initiatives of the Office of Disability Employment Policy (ODEP).

In the past year, ODEP has worked to ensure that the HS/HT program reflects the latest in evidence-based research on what youth with disabilities need to transition to employment successfully. HS/HT sites strive to deliver sites incorporating four design features into their programs: preparatory experiences, connecting activities, work-based experiences, and youth development and leadership activities.

Preparatory Experience

This design feature includes activities and services undertaken by youth at the program site or collaborating education site in accepting and nurturing environments that relate to career assessment (formal and informal), opportunity awareness, and work-readiness skills that includes learning about computers.

Connecting Activities (Program Linkages)

This feature examines the connecting activities necessary to assist participants' transition to their next phase in life - one that will hopefully provide for economic self-sufficiency. The focus is on services and activities requiring support from other organizations, such as tutoring to improve academic performance, assistive technology to address accommodation needs, mentoring, and transportation.

Work-Based Experiences

Work-based experiences include a range of activities that build up to on-the-job experiences. These include site visits, job shadowing, internships, entrepreneurial ventures, and paid employment. Such experiences are an essential component to promoting informed choice in high tech jobs.

Youth Development and Leadership

Youth development and leadership activities help young people become self-sufficient and productive members of society. This design feature includes providing supportive adults, developing independent decision-making skills, encouraging service learning, and promoting the development of self-determination and self-advocacy skills.

High School/High Tech programs depend on community involvement and require partnerships between many stakeholders, depending on the dynamics of the locality. The programs flourish when public/private partnerships develop around the design features. Suggested HS/HT partners include Workforce Investment Boards, Vocational Rehabilitation agencies, school systems, colleges and universities, disability service providers, employers, and families.

(Source: "High School/High Tech," U.S. Department of Labor (DOL))

Additional Competencies That Maximize Success among Youth with Disabilities

- Knowledge of what accommodations and supports, including assistive technology, one needs in education settings and how to use them
- Ability to self-advocate for accommodations and supports in education settings

CHAPTER 43
EDUCATIONAL OPTIONS AFTER HIGH SCHOOL

About This Chapter: "Educational Options after High School," © 2017 Omnigraphics. Reviewed July 2020.

Students with learning disabilities (LDs) have many options for continuing their education after high school, including four-year universities, two-year colleges, vocational or technical programs, adult basic education (ABE) or continuing education programs, and life skills training. The unique challenges of LD make it especially important for you to plan ahead, set goals, and stay organized as you consider your postsecondary education options. Planning for college can begin as early as your freshman year of high school. You should work with your teachers, guidance counselors, and Individual Education Plan (IEP) team to select courses that will help prepare you for success in college and in your transition to adulthood.

Planning for College
The process of planning for postsecondary education includes the following steps:
- **Identify your interests.** High school is an ideal time to identify your personal interests and explore possible career paths in those areas. School guidance counselors can provide you with various tools and assessments to help you find career options that fit your strengths and interests. You can also learn about potential careers by attending job fairs, talking with people who work in fields of interest to you, and volunteering or job shadowing.
- **Practice self-advocacy.** Self-advocacy means speaking up for yourself and taking more responsibility for the decisions affecting your life. Practicing self-advocacy in high school helps you gain the independence you will need in college. You can become a stronger self-advocate by understanding your disability and how it impacts your learning, and by asking for accommodations in a positive way. Once you reach college, these skills will

help you take responsibility for planning your future and accessing the support services you need to get there.

- **Improve your study habits.** Your success in college will depend on your ability to stay organized and use your time wisely. You will need to take responsibility for managing your class schedule, doing your homework, and using the study methods that work best for you. Working to develop strong study habits in high school gives you an advantage in making the transition to college.
- **Prepare for college entrance exams.** Students with LD are eligible for test-taking accommodations on the ACT and SAT college entrance exams. These tests are typically taken in the spring of your junior year of high school and in the fall of your senior year of high school. A variety of online and community resources are available to help students prepare and practice for these standardized tests.
- **Research schools and programs.** Your high school guidance counselor can provide a vast amount of information about postsecondary educational options. The key is to identify the schools and programs that best match your career interests and your academic abilities. Research the requirements for admission and graduation to see whether you meet them. You can also contact the disability services offices at various schools to inquire about the supports and accommodations they offer for students with LD.

Postsecondary Educational Options

Once you narrow down your career interests and future goals, you are ready to decide which type of postsecondary education option best fits your needs. The main choices include the following:

- **Four-year colleges and universities.** There are nearly 2,500 of these institutions in the United States. They can be public or private, and they vary by size, courses of study offered, admission requirements, and academic standards. Students who complete a degree program typically earn a bachelor's degree. Those who are interested in careers that require advanced training may also attend graduate or professional schools to earn a master's or doctoral degree.

- **Two-year community or junior colleges.** There are more than 1,000 of these institutions in the United States. Although they vary in size and can be public or private, most have easier admissions policies than larger universities and also tend to be less expensive. Students who complete a degree program typically earn an associate's or applied science degree. Some two-year degree programs prepare you for specific careers—such as accounting or criminal justice—while others allow you to earn credits that will transfer to a four-year college. Most public community colleges do not offer student housing, so they tend to serve people from the local community.
- **Vocational and technical schools.** These programs offer specialized training to prepare students for particular occupations, such as computer technician, plumber, broadcast technician, medical assistant, veterinary assistant, truck driver, or cosmetologist. They may be public or private.
- **Adult and continuing education programs.** Adult Basic Education (ABE) programs offer free tutoring and instruction in basic skills like reading, writing, and math for students who have not yet earned a high school diploma. Students can improve their literacy and academic skills in order to take the high-school equivalency exam. Continuing education classes can be found at many community colleges and some four-year universities. These courses have minimal admission standards and offer training in a variety of fields, such as marketing, technology, food management, and health services. Some students take continuing education courses to explore their personal interests, while others receive certification in specific fields.
- **Life skills training.** These programs offer training in social skills, life management skills, and independent living for students who may not be able to attend college or vocational programs.

In order to choose the best postsecondary educational option for you, it is important to investigate the level of support available for students with LD in each setting. Since it is a good idea to visit campuses, meet with representatives from the office of disability support services, and inquire whether the school or program will provide accommodations that meet your needs.

References

1. "At a Glance: Types of Colleges and How They Differ," Understood.org, 2016.
2. "Information for Students with Disabilities," EducationQuest, n.d.
3. "Postsecondary Educational Options," Learning Disabilities Association of America (LDA), 2017.
4. Stefanakos, Victoria Scanlan. "Planning for College: A Four-Year Guide for High School Students," Understood.org, 2016.

CHAPTER 44

PREPARING FOR POSTSECONDARY EDUCATION

About This Chapter: This chapter includes text excerpted from "Students with Disabilities Preparing for Postsecondary Education," U.S. Department of Education (ED), January 10, 2020.

Frequently Asked Questions

As a Student with a Disability Leaving High School and Entering Postsecondary Education, Will You See Differences in Your Rights and How They Are Addressed?

Yes. Section 504 and Title II protect elementary, secondary, and postsecondary students from discrimination. Nevertheless, several of the requirements that apply through high school are different from the requirements that apply beyond high school. For instance, Section 504 requires a school district to provide a free appropriate public education (FAPE) to each child with a disability in the district's jurisdiction. Whatever the disability, a school district must identify an individual's educational needs and provide any regular or special education and related aids and services necessary to meet those needs as well as it is meeting the needs of students without disabilities.

Unlike your high school, however, your postsecondary school is not required to provide FAPE. Rather, your postsecondary school is required to provide appropriate academic adjustments as necessary to ensure that it does not discriminate on the basis of disability. In addition, if your postsecondary school provides housing to non-disabled students, it must provide comparable, convenient, and accessible housing to students with disabilities at the same cost.

Other important differences that you need to know, even before you arrive at your postsecondary school, are addressed in the remaining questions.

May a Postsecondary School Deny Your Admission Because You Have a Disability?

No. If you meet the essential requirements for admission, a postsecondary school may not deny your admission simply because you have a disability.

Do You Have to Inform a Postsecondary School That You Have a Disability?

No. But, if you want the school to provide an academic adjustment, you must identify yourself as having a disability. Likewise, you should let the school know about your disability if you want to ensure that you are assigned to accessible facilities. In any event, your disclosure of a disability is always voluntary.

What Academic Adjustments Must a Postsecondary School Provide?

The appropriate academic adjustment must be determined based on your disability and individual needs. Academic adjustments may include auxiliary aids and services, as well as modifications to academic requirements as necessary to ensure equal educational opportunity. Examples of adjustments are: arranging for priority registration; reducing a course load; substituting one course for another; providing note takers, recording devices, sign language interpreters, extended time for testing, and, if telephones are provided in dorm rooms, a TTY in your dorm room; and equipping school computers with screen-reading, voice recognition, or other adaptive software or hardware.

In providing an academic adjustment, your postsecondary school is not required to lower or substantially modify essential requirements. For example, although your school may be required to provide extended testing time, it is not required to change the substantive content of the test. In addition, your postsecondary school does not have to make adjustments that would fundamentally alter the nature of a service, program, or activity, or that would result in an undue financial or administrative burden. Finally, your postsecondary school does not have to provide personal attendants, individually prescribed devices, readers for personal use or study, or other devices or services of a personal nature, such as tutoring and typing.

If You Want an Academic Adjustment, What Must You Do?

You must inform the school that you have a disability and need an academic adjustment. Unlike your school district, your postsecondary school is not required to identify you as having a disability or to assess your needs.

Your postsecondary school may require you to follow reasonable procedures to request an academic adjustment. You are responsible for knowing and following those procedures. In their publications providing general information, postsecondary schools usually include information on the procedures and contacts for requesting an academic adjustment. Such publications include recruitment materials, catalogs, and student handbooks, and are often available on school websites. Many schools also have staff whose purpose is to assist students with disabilities. If you are unable to locate the procedures, ask a school official, such as an admissions officer or counselor.

When Should You Request an Academic Adjustment?

Although you may request an academic adjustment from your postsecondary school at any time, you should request it as early as possible. Some academic adjustments may take more time to provide than others. You should follow your school's procedures to ensure that the school has enough time to review your request and provide an appropriate academic adjustment.

Do You Have to Prove That You Have a Disability to Obtain an Academic Adjustment?

Generally, yes. Your school will probably require you to provide documentation showing that you have a current disability and need an academic adjustment.

What Documentation Should You Provide?

Schools may set reasonable standards for documentation. Some schools require more documentation than others. They may require you to provide documentation prepared by an appropriate professional, such as a medical doctor, psychologist, or other qualified diagnosticians. The required documentation may include one or more of the following: a diagnosis of your current disability, as well as supporting information, such as the date of the diagnosis, how that diagnosis was reached, and the credentials of the diagnosing professional; information on how your disability affects a major life activity; and information on how the disability affects your academic performance. The documentation should provide enough information for you and your school to decide what is an appropriate academic adjustment.

An individualized education program (IEP) or Section 504 plan, if you have one, may help identify services that have been effective for you. This is generally not sufficient documentation, however, because of the differences between postsecondary education and high school education. What you need to meet the new demands of postsecondary education may be different from what worked for you in high school. Also, in some cases, the nature of a disability may change.

If the documentation that you have does not meet the postsecondary school's requirements, a school official should tell you in a timely manner what additional documentation you need to provide. You may need a new evaluation in order to provide the required documentation.

Who Has to Pay for a New Evaluation?

Neither your high school nor your postsecondary school is required to conduct or pay for a new evaluation to document your disability and need for an academic adjustment. You may, therefore, have to pay or find funding to pay an appropriate professional for an evaluation. If you are eligible for services through your state vocational rehabilitation agency, you may qualify for an evaluation at no cost to you. You may locate your state vocational rehabilitation agency at rsa.ed.gov by clicking on "Info about RSA," then "People and Offices," and then "State Agencies/Contacts."

Once the School Has Received the Necessary Documentation from You What Should You Expect?

To determine an appropriate academic adjustment, the school will review your request in light of the essential requirements for the relevant program. It is important to remember that the school is not required to lower or waive essential requirements. If you have requested a specific academic adjustment, the school may offer that academic adjustment, or it may offer an effective alternative. The school may also conduct its own evaluation of your disability and needs at its own expense.

You should expect your school to work with you in an interactive process to identify an appropriate academic adjustment. Unlike the experience you may have had in high school, however, do not expect your postsecondary school to invite your parents to participate in the process or to develop an IEP for you.

What If the Academic Adjustment the U.S. Department of Education Identified Is Not Working?

Let the school know as soon as you become aware that the results are not what you expected. It may be too late to correct the problem if you wait until the course or activity is completed. You and your school should work together to resolve the problem.

May a Postsecondary School Charge You for Providing an Academic Adjustment?

No. Nor may it charge students with disabilities more for participating in its programs or activities than it charges students who do not have disabilities.

What Can You Do If You Believe the School Is Discriminating against You?

Practically every postsecondary school must have a person—frequently called the "Section 504 Coordinator," "ADA Coordinator," or "Disability Services Coordinator"— who coordinates the school's compliance with Section 504, Title II, or both laws. You may contact that person for information about how to address your concerns.

The school must also have grievance procedures. These procedures are not the same as the due process procedures with which you may be familiar from high school. But, the postsecondary school's grievance procedures must include steps to ensure that you may raise your concerns fully and fairly, and must provide for the prompt and equitable resolution of complaints.

School publications, such as student handbooks and catalogs, usually describe the steps that you must take to start the grievance process. Often, schools have both formal and informal processes. If you decide to use a grievance process, you should be prepared to present all the reasons that support your request.

If you are dissatisfied with the outcome of the school's grievance procedures or wish to pursue an alternative to using those procedures, you may file a complaint against the school with OCR or in a court. You may learn more about the OCR complaint process from the brochure *How to File a Discrimination Complaint with the Office for Civil Rights*, which you may obtain by contacting us at the addresses and phone numbers below, or at www.ed.gov/ocr/docs/howto.html.

Customer Service Team
Office for Civil Rights (OCR)
U.S. Department of Education (ED)
Washington, DC 20202-1100
Toll-free: 800-421-3481
Toll-free TDD: 877-521-2172
E-mail: ocr@ed.gov
Website: www.ed.gov/ocr

If you would like more information about the responsibilities of postsecondary schools to students with disabilities, read the OCR brochure *Auxiliary Aids and Services for Postsecondary Students with Disabilities: Higher Education's Obligations Under Section 504 and Title II of the ADA*. You may obtain a copy at www.ed.gov/ocr/docs/auxaids.html.

Students with disabilities who know their rights and responsibilities are much better equipped to succeed in postsecondary school. The U.S. Department of Education encourages you to work with the staff at your school because they, too, want you to succeed. Seek the support of family, friends, and fellow students, including those with disabilities. Know your talents and capitalize on them, and believe in yourself as you embrace new challenges in your education.

CHAPTER 45
CONNECTING ACTIVITIES TO GAIN ACCESS TO CHOSEN POSTSCHOOL OPTIONS

About This Chapter: This chapter includes text excerpted from "Youth in Transition—Connecting Activities," U.S. Department of Labor (DOL), July 26, 2019.

Young people need to be connected to programs, services, activities, and supports that help them gain access to chosen postschool options. All youth may also need one or more of the following:

- Skills for navigating through the healthcare system to access medical, mental, behavioral, and reproductive health services
- Skills for self-care, healthcare decision making, and self-advocacy
- Ability to choose and engage in recreation and leisure activities that promote health and well-being
- Knowledge and skills to find, secure, and maintain safe, stable, and accessible housing
- Ability to secure reliable, accessible transportation (public or personal)
- Skills and confidence needed to travel independently throughout one's community
- Ability to secure sufficient nutritious food and recognition of the benefits of choosing healthy foods
- Knowledge and skills to secure quality childcare
- Ability to responsibly parent a child
- Ability to access contraception and sexual-health information
- Independent living and life skills
- Ability to manage financial resources effectively
- Ability to make decisions and develop a plan for continuing one's education and training, including pursuing postsecondary education and occupational credentials

- Knowledge about one's rights and ability to find and utilize legal and advocacy services appropriate to one's needs and age (e.g., services specific to English Language Learners (ELLs) and migrant youth, veterans, LGBT youth, court-involved youth, foster care youth, and those with mental-health challenges)

Additional Competencies That Maximize Success among Youth with Disabilities

- Ability to find and utilize disability-related services such as assistive technology, benefits counseling, and personal assistance services
- Ability to advocate for oneself and manage disability-related services

Education, Employment, and Independent Living

Being connected to programs, services, activities, information, and supports helps to maximize youth success. Learning about education, competitive integrated employment, and disability-related programs and services, helps youth become aware of their options and make informed choices. Areas of importance include civil rights, community life, education, emergency preparedness, employment, benefits, work incentives, health, housing, technology, and transportation.

The Workforce Innovation and Opportunity Act expands services to better support students and youth with disabilities in career development and transition planning. Title 1 of the Workforce Innovation and Opportunity Act (WIOA) (www.dol.gov/agencies/eta/wioa) authorizes the provision of career planning for eligible individuals. Career planning offers a person-centered approach to coordinate necessary support services before and after job placement.

At least 20 percent of local Title I Youth formula funds must be used for work experiences including:
- Summer and year-round employment opportunities
- Pre-apprenticeships
- Internships and job shadowing
- On-the-job training

Moreover, activities that help youth transition to postsecondary education and training are also explicitly included within the list of Title I Youth program elements (wdr.doleta.gov/directives/corr_doc.cfm?docn=4244).

Section 113 of the Rehabilitation Act, as amended by WIOA authorizes Vocational Rehabilitation agencies (rsa.ed.gov) to use federally reserved funds, and any funds made available to State, local, or private funding sources, to coordinate with local educational agencies to provide students with disabilities pre-employment transition services including the following required activities:
- Job exploration counseling
- Work-based learning experiences, which may include in school or after school opportunities, or experience outside the traditional school setting (including internships), that is provided in an integrated environment to the maximum extent possible
- Counseling on opportunities for enrollment in comprehensive transition or postsecondary educational programs at institutions of higher education
- Workplace readiness training to develop social skills and independent living

- Instruction in self-advocacy, (including instruction in person-centered planning), which may include peer mentoring

Substantial, coordinated, well-designed services can improve transition outcomes. Extensive collaborative partnerships are needed to ensure a "continuum of services" across agency boundaries. FPT partners have several examples of interagency activities, collaborative projects, and coordinated services that impact transition outcomes. These include the Social Security Administration's (SSA) Youth Transition Demonstration (YTD) (2006-2012) (www.ssa.gov/disabilityresearch/youth.htm), the Substance Abuse and Mental Health Services Administration's (SAMHSA) Health Transitions program (www.samhsa.gov/grants/grant-announcements/sm-14-017) and the U.S. Department of Education's (ED) National Technical Assistance Center (NTAC) on Improving Transition to Postsecondary Education and Employment for Students with Disabilities (www.transitionta.org). Given that no single agency can address all the transition needs of youth with disabilities, designing service delivery consistent with the Guideposts for Success (www.ncwd-youth.info/publications/guideposts) and other similar frameworks can help to ensure that youth receive the services and supports they need to succeed.

Education and Training systems for preparing low-skilled youth with disabilities for marketable jobs can be complex and difficult to navigate. Career pathways (careertech.org/sites/default/files/Joint_Letter_Career_Pathways.pdf) offer an efficient and customer-centered approach to training and education. This approach integrates the educational instruction, workforce development, and human and social services and supports that are linked to labor market trends and employer needs, leading to stackable credentials.

(Source: "Youth in Transition—Federal Partners in Transition," U.S. Department of Labor (DOL))

PART 6 | CAREER OPTIONS AND EMPLOYMENT SUPPORT

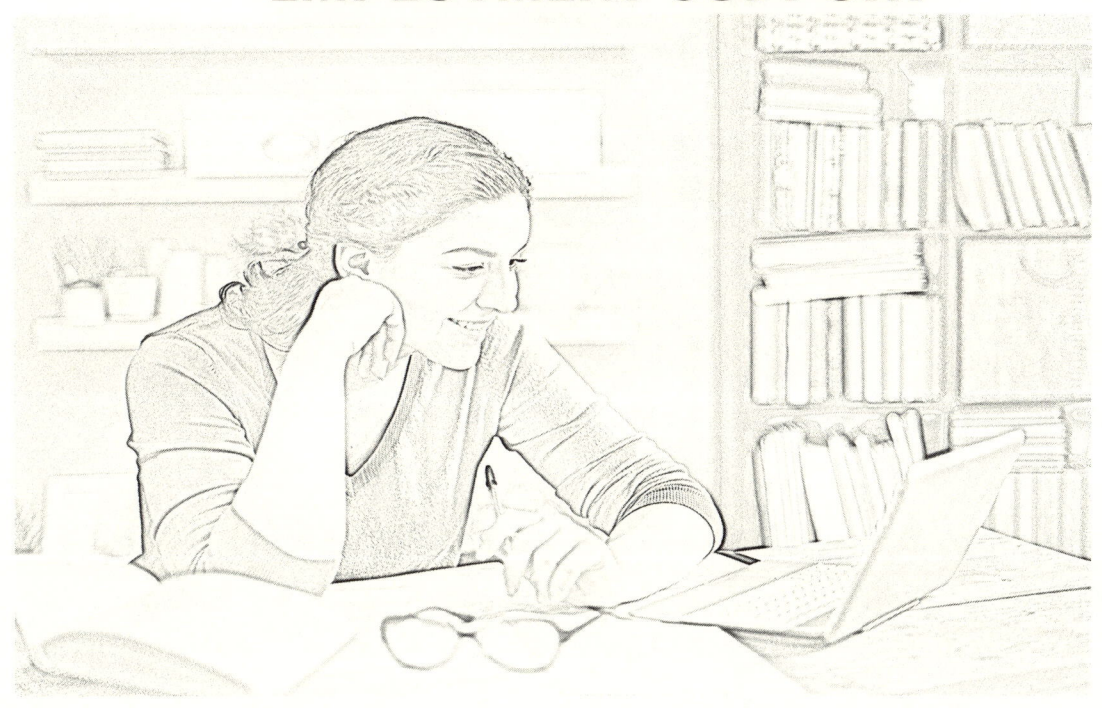

CHAPTER 46
TRANSITION PLANNING

About This Chapter: This chapter includes text excerpted from "Youth with Disabilities—Strategies and Resources," Youth.gov, October 3, 2012. Reviewed July 2020.

Transition Planning for Youth and Young Adults with Disabilities

Because successful transition planning for youth and young adults with disabilities should begin well before the student reaches "transition age," and should ideally involve multiple parties and agencies, the process may be especially complex. Effective communication and collaboration between key agencies is essential.

Transition activities need to be coordinated, youth-focused, and results-oriented, addressing needs in the areas of:

- Employment
- High school graduation and dropout prevention
- Postsecondary education
- Vocational education
- Healthcare
- Community and civic engagement
- Relationships with friends and family
- Daily living skills
- Housing

Considerations for Transition Planning for Youth in Juvenile Justice and Foster Care

Planning for post-high school experiences for students who have disabilities and who are also involved with the juvenile justice system requires not only consideration of the student's interests and strengths—as required by IDEA 2004—but also a comprehensive and coordinated approach that supports the student's educational development in the context of developing skills for successful community living and possibly navigating the justice system. The National Evaluation and Technical Assistance Center for the Education of Children and Youth who are neglected, delinquent, or at-risk (neglected-delinquent.ed.gov) recommends family-driven, youth-guided collaborative planning in which "performance and outcomes must be monitored through an established plan with the responsibility for the assessment being assigned to either an education liaison or volunteer mentors."

Transition planning for youth and young adults with disabilities who are in foster care should begin as early as possible and no later than age 16. Working closely with the Individual Education Plan (IEP) team and connecting to federal programs designed to support transition to adulthood, foster care youth can chart a successful course toward post-high school education, employment, and independent living.

Key Elements of Successful Transition Plans

A key goal of transition planning is not just to "transition out" into the community, but also to focus on helping the young person thrive and flourish as an adult, with the wide range of skills and activities that adult living requires. Planning involves careful consideration of available resources (such as social security disability benefits, health insurance, Medicaid, assistive technology grants, funding for housing, etc.), as well as navigation of information and services provided by multiple organizations and agencies, such as:

- Independent living centers
- Employment agencies
- One-stop centers
- Postsecondary education providers
- Recreation centers
- The U.S. Department of Labor's (DOL) Office of Disability Employment
- Vocational rehabilitation services
- Assistive technology centers
- Young adult advocacy organizations, such as Youth MOVE

Though there are many components of a successful transition plan, key areas to focus on include self-advocacy/self-determination, postsecondary education and training, employment, and community living.

Self-Advocacy/Self-Determination

The most critical consideration of the IEP and transition planning process is the involvement and engagement of the youth or young adult. This ensures both that her or his needs, interests, and desires are represented, and that the youth gains or practices necessary skills in self-advocacy. Youth and young adults who do not have disabilities plan and dream about the future, are usually agents in their own destinies. Wherever possible, students with disabilities should have the same opportunities for self-determination in planning their lives, and expressing their wishes and hopes for the future. Participation in planning enables youth and young adults with disabilities to gain valuable experience with goal setting, locating resources and support, and advocating for themselves within their community. These experiences are critical for success beyond the classroom, and are an important component of transition planning. Research demonstrates a connection between student self-advocacy and improved academic and postschool outcomes; therefore, students with disabilities should be encouraged and empowered to participate actively and even to lead the development of their IEPs.

Postsecondary Education and Training

As schools work to develop "College and Career-Ready Students," an emphasis on preparation for postsecondary education and employment should shape transition planning. When a student with a disability completes high school with a regular high school diploma, the school district is required to provide the student with a Summary of Performance (SOP).

The purpose of the SOP is to provide information to postsecondary education institutions and to prospective employers on the young adult's capabilities, strengths, and skills as demonstrated in high school, as well as a description of the types of supports that contributed to successful performance as a student, and recommendations on how to assist in meeting her or his postsecondary goals. The SOP is not, itself, documentation of eligibility for services or programs. It may, however, include information that will assist those making future eligibility determinations. Effective transition planning practices can include a student-developed SOP, which reflects the student's own description of her or his high school accomplishments and the support needed to reach postsecondary goal(s). While it is the school district's responsibility to provide an SOP to the student, students can benefit from direct involvement in understanding and articulating ways in which they can meet their postschool goals.

Employment

Because many people with disabilities may at some point be unemployed or underemployed, or may face discrimination in the workplace, a transition plan that addresses employment needs, necessary supports, and skill development is essential. This may include curricula that address workplace culture and routines, job placement assistance, apprenticeships, and skills needed for interviewing, as well as rights in the workplace under the Americans with Disabilities Act. Supported employment in the form of job coaches, job development, training, transportation, and assistive technology can help youth with disabilities find and maintain jobs.

Community Living

Often, transition planning teams focus primarily on employment options and neglect to consider skills necessary for youth with disabilities to become active and productive members of their communities. Finding friends, enjoying leisure activities, and participating in community events should all be considered key components of transition planning. Depending on a student's interests and needs, these could include field trips (both virtually and in person) to various community locations, agencies, and recreation centers. Teams may also consider adaptive devices, equipment, and technologies that can help the young person achieve a healthy lifestyle and participate in recreational activities.

CHAPTER 47
LEARNING ABOUT CAREER OPTIONS

About This Chapter: Text under the heading "Career Preparation and Work-Based Learning Experiences" is excerpted from "Youth in Transition—Career Preparation and Work-Based Learning Experiences," U.S. Department of Labor (DOL), July 25, 2019; Text beginning with the heading "Mentoring" is excerpted from "Career Exploration and Skill Development," Youth.gov, October 16, 2016. Reviewed July 2020.

Career Preparation and Work-Based Learning Experiences

Career preparation and work-based learning experiences are essential in order to form and develop aspirations and to make informed choices about careers. These experiences can be provided during the school day, or through after-school programs, and will require collaborations with other organizations. All youth need information on career options, including:

- Understanding of the role that employment plays in economic self-sufficiency and the motivation to build skills, explore careers, and seek employment to live the life a youth desires
- Self-exploration skills that enable youth to identify interests, skills, and values
- Career exploration skills that enable youth to identify how various career options match their interests, skills, and work preferences
- Ability to make informed choices about their long-term career interests and the corresponding secondary and postsecondary coursework and industry-recognized credentials necessary to pursue these interests
- Career-specific work skills and knowledge as well as employability or "soft" skills such as communication, leadership, decision-making, and conflict management skills
- Career planning and management skills, including academic planning, decision-making related to postsecondary pathways, career readiness skills, job search skills, and financial literacy

Additional Competencies That Maximize Success among Youth with Disabilities

- Knowledge of what accommodations and supports, including assistive technology, one needs in the workplace and training settings and how to use them
- Ability to self-advocate for accommodations and supports in the workplace and training settings

Mentoring

Mentoring—matching youth or "mentees" with responsible, caring "mentors," usually adults—has been found to be an important support for youth as they transition to adulthood and the workforce. Mentoring provides opportunities for youth to develop emotional bonds with mentors who have more life experience and can provide support, guidance, and opportunities to help them succeed in life and meet their goals.

Mentoring relationships can be formal or informal, with substantial variation, but the essential components include creating caring, empathetic, consistent, and long-lasting relationships, often with some combination of role modeling, teaching, and advising. One form of mentoring, called "instrumental" or "topic-focused mentoring," focuses on a particular problem and aims at helping mentees reach specific goals, such as improving academic performance or preparing for employment opportunities.

Career-focused mentoring, a type of instrumental or topic-focused mentoring, can take a variety of forms and may focus on different pieces of career development and employment. Some examples include assisting with the following:

- Writing resumes and cover letters
- Conducting mock interviews and providing support for answering interview questions
- Exploring possible careers and assisting with job, internship, or program searches
- Developing on-the-job skills (soft skills or technical skills)
- Modeling behavior, attitudes, or skills in the workplace (job shadowing)
- Career planning and goal setting

Apprenticeships and internships can provide on-the-job opportunities to integrate mentoring into employment experiences for youth.

Assessment, Testing, and Counseling

Self-assessments help teach youth about themselves so that they can find a career that is a good fit for their interests and skills. They allow youth to explore:

- What they do and do not like
- How they react to certain situations
- Their skills
- Values

A professional, such as a counselor at a high school, trade or vocational school, college, or career training center, can help in selecting an appropriate assessment, interpreting the results, and providing career counseling.

The U.S. Department of Labor (DOL), Employment and Training Administration (ETA) sponsors two valuable resources to assist youth identify career pathways. CareerOneStop (www.careeronestop.org) is a website that provides a range of career-exploration help.

- Up-do-date information on job salary and benefit information and related education and training opportunities
- Job search tools, resumes, and interview resources, and people and places to help jobseekers virtually, such as *What's My Next Move* (www. mynextmove.org), a guide to exploring careers for youth

The American Job Centers (AJCs), also known as "One Stop Centers," provide job referrals, counseling, and other supportive services to help with both job search and location of training and education resources. AJCs have locations (www.careerone-stop.org/LocalHelp/AmericanJobCenters/find-american-job-centers.aspx) across the United States.

The National Collaborative on Workforce and Disability (www.ncwd-youth.info/topic/assessment) provides a range of assessments that can help with the transition from school to employment. In addition to their focus on career planning, these resources recognize unique challenges faced by students with disabilities.

An additional online resource, Students and Career Advisors (careeronestop.org/StudentsandCareerAdvisors/StudentsandCareerAdvisors.aspx), allows students, career advisors, and parents to learn more about potential career opportunities. This resource provides opportunities for students to explore their interests, learn about potential careers, learn how to get job experience, and find additional educational opportunities to support career development.

Individualized Learning Plans

The goal of an Individualized Learning Plan (ILP), also known as "Individual Service Strategy" (ISS), is to connect what youth are doing in the classroom with their career and college goals and aspirations. ILPs help youth discover their skills and interests, match their interests with degrees and careers, set goals, and follow through in a thoughtful and meaningful way.

Job Search Assistance

Finding available jobs can be difficult. It is important for youth to recognize that finding a job often takes time and it is important to develop a plan, schedule, and goals when conducting a search. Many sources list available jobs, from newspapers to listservs to online directories. CareerOneStop (www.careeronestop.org) has online job listings that provide information, and knowledgeable staff at its AJCs are available to assist with counseling youth on various employment options. Tools such as GetMyFuture (www.careeronestop.org/GetMyFuture/default.aspx), which allows youth to search for career opportunities based on past employment experiences, can help young people identify future careers that may be available based on their previous work experience. College career centers, CareerOneStop, and AJCs can help youth prepare their resumes, write cover letters, and practice interviewing. State vocational rehabilitation agencies are typically represented at or can be accessed through AJCs to provide assistance for youth with disabilities in the job search process. College career centers can also provide valuable resources for students as they search for jobs and internships.

Soft and Technical Skill Development and Training

Soft skills are generally defined as personal qualities, not technical, that translate to good job performance. They have been named by employers to be most important for successful job performance. Soft skills can be learned through a variety of means, including classroom instruction, youth programs, volunteering, and service-learning.

More than 50 percent of manufacturers who completed the 2005 skills gap survey reported that technical skills will play an important role in meeting the needs of employers in the upcoming years. Vocational training courses or work-study programs can teach marketable technical or occupational skills. CareerOneStop (www.careeronestop.org) and AJCs can make referrals to local postsecondary institutions and youth-serving agencies when training and other services are needed. Not only are the people there knowledgeable about these resources, but they also can approve vouchers to defray training costs. The Center for Employment Training (CET) (cetweb.org) is a nonprofit organization that has partnerships with the DOL. CET has pioneered the practice of open-ended, competency-based training that uses the workplace as the context for simulations. The individualized training allows youth to train at their own pace and explore career options firsthand. The majority of training is provided through hands-on experience. The Office of Vocational and Adult Education (OVAE) (www2.ed.gov/about/offices/list/ovae/index.html) within the U.S. Department of Education (ED) also helps states, schools, and community colleges support technical and vocational education.

Apprenticeships

Youth apprenticeship programs grew out of the school-to-work movement and offer youth classroom instruction combined with structured on-the-job training with a mentor. The training is split between academic courses and vocational training, while on-the-job portion provides opportunities for practice in and understanding of work-based contexts for classroom instruction.

Youth apprenticeships may lead to admission to adult registered apprenticeship programs after graduation. The DOL (www.dol.gov/apprenticeship) sponsors registered apprenticeship programs that meet its standards. The minimum requirement for participation in a registered apprenticeship program may vary by the skills demanded for the program, but to be eligible, youth must be at least 16. Because of restrictions, some hazardous jobs are limited to individuals over 18. Participation in apprenticeships allows youth to receive the following:

- **A paycheck.** From day one, youth earn a paycheck guaranteed to increase over time as they acquire new skills.
- **Hands-on career training.** Apprentices receive practical on-the-job learning in a wide selection of programs, such as healthcare, construction, information technology, and geospatial careers.
- **An education.** Apprentices receive hands-on learning and related instruction to supplement the hand-on-learning and have the potential to earn college credit, even an associate's or bachelor's degree, in many cases paid for by the employer.
- **A career.** Once the apprenticeship is completed, youth are on their way to successful long-term careers with competitive salaries and little or no educational debt.
- **National industry certification.** When an apprentice completes a Registered Apprenticeship program, she or he will be certified and can take that certification anywhere in the United States.
- **The opportunity to work with recognizable partners.** Many of the nation's most recognizable companies, such as CVS Health and UPS, have Registered Apprenticeship programs.

The Office of Disability Employment Policy (ODEP) (www.dol.gov/odep/topics/youth/Apprenticeship.htm) provides a toolkit and other resources to increase the capacity of programs to provide integrated inclusive apprenticeship training to youth and young adults with a full range of disabilities, including those with the most significant disabilities. ODEP also provides guidance on how to use the increased flexibilities in the DOL apprenticeship regulations.

Internships

Internships, both paid and unpaid, provide youth with short-term, practical experiences to learn about careers, develop networks, and experience the workplace. The Wage and Hour Division (WHD) at the DOL has identified six criteria (www.dol.gov/sites/dolgov/files/WHD/legacy/files/whdfs71.pdf) to help determine whether interns must be paid the minimum wage and overtime under the Fair Labor Standards Act. Internships are available in a diverse array of career fields and can be formal or informal. Internships give youth the opportunity to explore what they like and do not like about certain careers. They allow youth who might not know what career they want to pursue with a chance to see whether a certain environment, job, or management style fits their needs. Both on-the-job experience and the application process allow youth to develop skills so that they are able to enter the job market with relevant career experience. According to a 2005 survey by the National Association of Colleges and Employers, 60 percent of employers hire college graduates who had completed internships. Further, on average more than half the students who completed internships were offered full-time positions upon internship completion.

CHAPTER 48
YOUTH DEVELOPMENT AND LEADERSHIP

About This Chapter: Text in this chapter begins with excerpts from "Youth in Transition—Youth Development and Leadership," U.S. Department of Labor (DOL), February 9, 2012. Reviewed July 2020; Text under the heading "Positive Youth Development" is excerpted from "Positive Youth Development," Youth.gov, February 4, 2017; Text under the heading "Leadership Training and Leadership Opportunities" is excerpted from "Youth Transitioning to Adulthood—Challenges," Youth.gov, October 3, 2012. Reviewed July 2020; Text under the heading "Promising Approaches" is excerpted from "Youth Transitioning to Adulthood—Promising Approaches," Youth.gov, October 3, 2012. Reviewed July 2020.

Youth development is a process that prepares young people to meet the challenges of adolescence and adulthood through a coordinated, progressive series of activities and experiences which help them gain skills and competencies. Youth leadership is part of that process. In order to control and direct their own lives based on informed decisions, all youth need the following:

- Self-efficacy or belief in one's capabilities
- Self-determination skills, knowledge, and beliefs that enable a person to engage in goal-directed, self-regulated, autonomous behaviors
- Agency or the ability to make choices about and take an active role in one's life path
- Interpersonal skills
- Critical thinking skills
- Self-advocacy skills including knowledge of self, knowledge of civil rights, communication, and leadership
- Leadership skills and initiative

Additional competencies that maximize success among youth with disabilities:
- Knowledge of if, when, and how to disclose, including an understanding of disability history, culture, and disability public policy as well as their rights and responsibilities

- Knowledge of oneself and sense of identity related to having a disability, including knowledge of one's strengths and what accommodations and supports enable participation and success in various situations
- Ability to effectively self-advocate for accommodations and supports in various settings including in educational, work, social, recreation, community, and other developmental contexts

Positive Youth Development

Based on the literature, the Interagency Working Group on Youth Programs (youth. gov/about-us), a collaboration of 21 federal departments and agencies that support youth, has created the following definition of positive youth development (PYD):

- Positive youth development (PYD) is an intentional, prosocial approach that engages youth within their communities, schools, organizations, peer groups, and families in a manner that is productive and constructive; recognizes, utilizes, and enhances young people's strengths; and promotes positive outcomes for young people by providing opportunities, fostering positive relationships, and furnishing the support needed to build on their leadership strengths.

The Interagency Working Group on Youth Programs developed a research agenda focused on positive youth development. Through a collaborative consensus-building process, representatives from federal agencies identified three research domains (conceptual issues, data sources and indicators, and program implementation and effectiveness) and key research questions that could benefit from future research.

Positive youth development (PYD) has its origins in the field of prevention. In the past, prevention efforts typically focused on single problems before they surfaced in youth, such as teen pregnancy, substance abuse, and juvenile delinquency.

Over time, practitioners, policymakers, funders, and researchers determined that promoting positive asset building and considering young people as resources were critical strategies. As a result, the youth development field began examining the role of resiliency—the protective factors in a young person's environment—and how these factors could influence one's ability to overcome adversity. Those factors included, but were not limited to, family support and monitoring; caring adults; positive peer groups; strong sense of self, self-esteem, and future aspirations; and engagement in school and community activities.

Researchers and practitioners began to report that young people who possess a diverse set of protective factors can, in fact, experience more positive outcomes. These findings encouraged the development of interventions and programs that reduce risks and strengthen protective factors. The programs and interventions are strengthened when they involve and engage youth as equal partners, ultimately providing benefits for both for the program and the involved youth.

Leadership Training and Leadership Opportunities

Leadership training and leadership opportunities are two key elements that can support successful youth development and transition to adulthood, but it often requires time and effort on the part of adults and programs, and therefore, is not always included in transition planning.

For leadership opportunities to be successful for youth and programs, the goals of youth involvement and roles that the youth will play need to be clearly defined. When this does not occur, it may result in negative experiences for both youth and adults.

Another challenge is that youth leaders often move on to new opportunities as they transition into adulthood and the workforce. If sustainability and succession planning strategies are not well developed, this can cause problems for programs as there is a continuous need to fill gaps when a youth moves on.

Adults may also be reluctant to provide youth with early leadership opportunities because of negative associations with teenagers, a lack of trust, or viewing youth as unable to take on a leadership role. Removing negative attitudes surrounding teens in leadership roles is critical, as these roles provide valuable skills and development opportunities necessary for successful transitions to adulthood.

Promising Approaches

Youth can be involved in leadership opportunities in their schools and communities. Some examples of opportunities for youth leadership include:

- Clubs, sports, and extracurricular activities
- Service-learning opportunities
- Volunteer programs
- School councils or student body leadership roles
- Leadership councils or youth boards for state and local government, among others

Through exploring activities such as service-learning, career opportunities, community participation, peer mentoring, and civic engagement, youth gain valuable experience in goal-setting, conflict resolution, problem-solving, and decision-making.

Youth development workers can help to address some of the challenges of involving youth in leadership roles by providing supportive, engaging opportunities that have clear roles and responsibilities, and established plans for sustainability. Adult service providers, educators, community members, and others can help young people develop leadership skills and build networks through the following:

- Encouraging partnerships between youth and their communities
- Providing opportunities for skill development and learning
- Ensuring that youth are active agents and helping them develop self-advocacy skills by placing youth in challenging situations where they need to use problem-solving skills to manage different risk factors

- Creating a supportive environment for youth that includes positive role models, constructive support, and mentoring
- Establishing cooperative, collaborative, and comprehensive transition plans that promote skill-building, leadership training, workforce development, partnerships, and engagement

CHAPTER 49
VOCATIONAL REHABILITATION

About This Chapter: This chapter includes text excerpted from "Employment Disability 101: Lesson One," U.S. Department of Education (ED), August 21, 2006. Reviewed July 2020.

The vocational rehabilitation (VR) program is a strong state-federal partnership that promotes the employment and independence of people with disabilities. The VR program, which began more than 85 years ago, was the first federally authorized program specifically created to serve the employment needs of people with physical disabilities not injured as a result of military service. Today, on average, more than 200,000 people with disabilities find employment each year with the help of the VR programs in their states.

The VR counselors have extensive specialized training, making them uniquely qualified to work with your business to:

- Identify qualified people with disabilities ready for employment
- Develop productive partnerships between your business and training organizations that support a person's career development while meeting your need for qualified applicants and skilled workers
- Provide access to cutting-edge assistive technologies that can improve the overall work performance of people with disabilities
- Provide information regarding the Americans with Disabilities Act (ADA) of 1990 and the Rehabilitation Act of 1973, as amended

Vocational rehabilitation counselors also have long-standing relationships with a wide variety of employers in your area. Some of the country's most successful businesses, such as SunTrust Bank, Starbucks and Manpower, Inc., to name a few, have thriving relationships with VR programs and counselors in their states that help them actively recruit, hire, support, and retain qualified workers with disabilities.

> ## VR100 Anniversary: Celebrating a Century of Success
>
> June 2, 2020, marked the 100th anniversary of the VR program. Office of Special Education and Rehabilitative Services' (OSERS) Rehabilitation Services Administration (RSA) paid tribute to this historical occasion by showcasing how the VR program helped change the lives of students and adults with disabilities!
>
> This year marks the 100th anniversary of the first federally funded program to assist people with disabilities who had not acquired their disabilities as a result of serving in the military.
>
> President Woodrow Wilson signed the Smith-Fess Act of 1920, also known as the "Industrial Rehabilitation Act" and referred to as "The National Civilian Vocational Rehabilitation Act," into law June 2, 1920.
>
> "The RSA plays a key leadership role through its resources and technical assistance to state vocational rehabilitation programs and others," said Mark Schultz, the OSERS RSA commissioner and delegated the authority to perform the functions and duties of the Assistant Secretary for OSERS. "Those 100 years of experience bring a responsibility of leadership on issues that impact the ability of individuals with disabilities to be employed and live independently."
>
> *(Source: "Vocational Rehabilitation—100 Years Later," U.S. Department of Education (ED))*

Note: The Civilian Vocational Rehabilitation Act, passed by Congress in 1920, defined vocational rehabilitation (VR) as a program for persons with physical disabilities. Mental disabilities were not part of the VR program until 1943.

Vocational Rehabilitation Puts Dreams within Reach

Vocational rehabilitation gave Kevin the help he needed for a promising future in medical technology. Through assistance from the Arkansas Rehabilitation Services, Kevin graduated with honors from the Oregon Institute of Technology with a degree in radiologic science-nuclear medicine technology. He passed the related national boards examination and is now licensed in nuclear medicine technology. He has a new job that pays $37 an hour.

Jeff was injured on his plumbing job several years before he contacted the state vocational rehabilitation agency. With VR's assistance, Jeff enrolled in accounting courses at his local community college. VR also provided adapted equipment that he would need for his new job as a teller and loan officer. Jeff has since been promoted and is now an assistant vice president of a bank in his hometown.

The findings of a recent longitudinal study, conducted by the U.S. Department of Education (ED) of 8,500 applicants and recipients of RSA's VR services, show that people with disabilities who have achieved competitive employment through existing business and VR partnerships have a nearly 85 percent job-retention rate after one year (2003). These findings concur with those of companies such as DuPont and Sears who have measured retention rates of their employees.

State vocational rehabilitation agencies help employ individuals with disabilities. To that end, VR agencies (with the support of their federal partners) stand ready to provide employers with qualified job candidates with disabilities to meet the workforce needs of American businesses. To connect to the single point of contact in a given state whose job it is to build and maintain employer relationships, visit the State Employment Specialists in Vocational Education's website at www.ed.gov/rschstat/research/pubs/vrpractices/busdev.html#al. In addition, you can find examples of how some state VR agencies approach their relationships with businesses.

CHAPTER 50
DISCLOSING DISABILITIES

About This Chapter: This chapter includes text excerpted from "Youth, Disclosure, and the Workplace Why, When, What, and How," U.S. Department of Labor (DOL), June 6, 2007. Reviewed July 2020.

Every job seeker with a disability is faced with the same decision: "Should I or should not I disclose my disability?" This decision may be framed differently depending upon whether you have a visible disability or a nonvisible disability. Ultimately, the decision of whether to disclose is entirely up to you.

Why Disclose in the Workplace

When you leave school and enter the workforce, many aspects of your life change. Among the many differences, is the requirement to share information about your disability if you want your employer to provide you with reasonable accommodations. In school, if you had an individualized education program (IEP), as required under the Individuals with Disabilities Education Act (IDEA), information about your disability and the accommodations you needed followed you from grade to grade. When you enter the workforce, the IDEA no longer applies to you. Instead, the Americans with Disabilities Act (ADA) and the Rehabilitation Act protect you from disability-related discrimination and provide for meaningful access. The laws require that qualified applicants and employees with disabilities be provided with reasonable accommodations. Yet, in order to benefit from the ADA and the Rehabilitation Act, you must disclose your disability. An employer is only required to provide work-related accommodations if you disclose your disability to the appropriate individuals.

When to Disclose Your Disability

There is no one "right" time or place to disclose your disability. Select a confidential place in which to disclose, and allow enough time for the person to ask questions. Do not dwell on the limitations of your disability. You should weigh the pros and cons of disclosure at each point of the job search, recruitment, and hiring process and make the decision to discuss your disability when it is appropriate for you. Consider the following stages:

- In a letter of application or cover letter
- Before an interview
- At the interview
- In a third-party phone call or reference
- Before any drug testing for illegal drugs
- After you have a job offer
- During your course of employment
- Never

How to Disclose Your Disability

Preparation is essential for disclosing your disability. Effective disclosure requires that you discuss your needs, and that you provide practical suggestions for reasonable job accommodations, if they are needed. One way to become comfortable with discussing your disability is to find someone you trust and practice the disclosure discussion with that person. The two of you can put together a disclosure script. It should contain relevant disability information and weave in your strengths. Always keep it positive!

What to Disclose about Your Disability

There is no required information to share about your disability. In fact, it will be different for everyone. For example, if you have an apparent disability it is often beneficial to address how you plan to accomplish tasks required by the job. This can affirm to the employer that you are suited for the position. Additionally, by demonstrating your own ease and comfort with the job requirements, you can relay to employers other traits that are desirable in an applicant. A person with a hidden disability, on the other hand, will first need to decide whether to disclose the disability, and subsequently determine what information to share about the disability. Generally, if you choose to disclose, it is most helpful to share the following:

- General information about your disability
- Why you are disclosing your disability
- How your disability affects your ability to perform key job tasks
- Types of accommodations that have worked for you in the past
- Types of accommodations you anticipate needing in the workplace

To Whom to Disclose Your Disability

Disclose your disability on a "need-to-know" basis. Provide further details about your disability as it applies to your work-related accommodations to the individual who has the authority to facilitate your accommodation request. Consider disclosing to the supervisor responsible for the hiring, promoting, and/or firing of employees. This person needs to be informed of your disability-related needs to provide the necessary support and judge your job performance fairly.

Disclosure Protections and Responsibilities

As a person with a disability, you have disclosure protections as well as significant responsibilities to yourself and to your employers.

You are entitled to:

- Have information about your disability treated confidentially and respectfully
- Seek information about hiring practices from any organization
- Choose to disclose your disability at any time during the employment process
- Receive reasonable accommodations for an interview
- Be considered for a position based on your skill and merit
- Have respectful questioning about your disability for the purpose of determining whether you need accommodations and if so, what kind

You have the responsibility to:

- Disclose your need for any work-related reasonable accommodations
- Bring your skills and merits to the table
- Be truthful, self-determined, and proactive

CHAPTER 51
LEARNING DISABILITIES ON THE JOB

Learning disabilities (LDs) can affect the work life of a teenager since they usually have constant trouble getting and maintaining employment without the proper training required to overcome their LD. Teenagers with LD experience an increase in the rate of unemployment and underemployment, as well as lower wages, lesser work hours, and annual income when compared to their nondisabled peers. There are five major reasons for challenges experienced on the job for teens with LD according to the National Center for Learning Disabilities (NCLD):

- **Efficiency.** Slow pace of work and having trouble with organizing things.
- **Time management.** Struggling with punctuality, planning, and meeting deadlines.
- **Accuracy.** Prone to making mistakes with reading tasks or writing correspondence.
- **Consecutive tasks.** Difficulty following a set of instructions to complete a complex task.
- **Social skills.** Problems with professional interactions and discussing how LD can affect the task they have been assigned.

These are a few of the common issues that lower the success rate of teenagers with LD, most of whom also have trouble with self-determination and empowerment skills.

Learning Disabilities and Work Opportunities

People with a learning disability may include one person who has difficulty reading, writing, and spelling things; whereas another person may have problems with math, speaking, thinking, and listening. Since learning disabilities are varied and complicated, it is often overlooked as a form of disability. Common LD conditions such as dyslexia and attention deficit hyperactivity disorder (ADHD) can make it quite challenging to create a successful career. However, these challenges should not hold back a person from exploring their talents. Humanity's greatest contributors such as Albert Einstein and Leonardo da Vinci are thought to have learning disabilities as well.

Americans with Disabilities Act

All U.S. citizens are protected by the Americans with Disabilities Act (ADA), which prevents discrimination in the workplace against people with disabilities. Discrimination charges can be filed through the U.S. Equal Employment Opportunity Commission (EEOC). This should be done within 180 days from the time of the alleged discrimination, but a few states allow up to 300 days before a complaint can be filed. However, revealing the learning disability is a matter of personal choice and solely the decision of the teenager. The EEOC has ruled that a person can disclose a disability at any time, from the first day of application till termination.

Accommodations for Employees with Learning Disability

Methods, strategies, techniques, and workplace adaptations that enable a person with a disability to perform their job are known as "accommodations." Reasonable accommodations are required as outlined by the ADA law, meaning they should not cause the employer undue hardships such as very high expenses or safety hazards. To be eligible for job accommodations, the disability should be disclosed to the employer by providing official documentation proving your learning disability or attention deficit disorder (ADD). There are various types of accommodations, depending on the kind of LD a person has and being aware of their specific accommodations needs can be of great help in the workplace.

Accommodations for teens with LD can be decided based on their limitations. The degree of limitations varies among people and a person rarely develops all of them. Also, some people with LD are able to perform their jobs without any such accommodations. The following is a list of possible limitations and work-related functions along with their equivalent accommodations:

Limitations

- **Executive functioning deficits**—flexible work schedule, noise-canceling headsets, on-site mentoring, etc.
- **Time management**—electronic organizers, additional time, training refreshers, etc.
- **Mathematics**—counting/measuring aids, talking calculators and cash register, modified written materials, etc.
- **Memory loss**—break reminder software, medication reminders, voice recorders, timers, etc.
- **Planning/prioritizing**—recorded directives and messages, organization/workflow management software, etc.
- **Reading**—color-coded manuals, outlines, and maps, screen magnification and screen reading software, verbal direction, etc.

- **Writing/spelling**—word processing software, writing aids, speech recognition software, etc.

Work-Related Function
- **Communication**—behavior modification techniques, assistant/attendant, etc.
- **Stress**—counseling/therapy, support person, remote work option, etc.
- **Cognitive function**—job coaches, training modifications, color-coded system, etc.

First-Time Job Recommendations for Teens with LD

Teens with LD can build up their confidence and self-esteem by landing a successful first job. It is essential to find a job that works well with their strengths or areas of expertise. A few common first-time jobs suitable for teens with LD include:

1. **Animal care.** This might be a perfect job for animal lovers, and it also focuses their attention, making the most of their energy and enthusiasm. Teens with language and speaking difficulties may find this job comfortable. It gives them an opportunity to help out in shelters and kennels and includes manual tasks such as hauling supplies and feeding or walking the animals.

2. **Landscaping or car wash.** Landscaping is a suitable work for teens with language problems as it involves manual labor and does not require much conversation. Teens with attention deficiency and executive function issues are suited for car washing since it gives them the quick satisfaction of finishing a job every few minutes. It can help them stay attentive and working for tips also gives them an incentive to stay focused on the task.

3. **Retail or restaurant.** Teens who are good with people can help with customer service at retail stores. They can also assist with shelving goods, bagging groceries, or use their artistic talents to create store displays. In restaurants, teens with LD/ADD have the opportunity to work as a team helping with food prep, dishwashing, floor mopping, and table busing. It can help them learn the basics of foodservice and keep them focused.

4. **Recreation assistant or pool maintenance.** For athletic teens, the local recreation center or the pool may be the perfect place to get a hands-on and active job opportunity during the summer. This can be of help for teens with attention deficiency, executive functioning, and reading issues. Recreation assistant jobs involve playing on the field, keeping kids busy, and hauling equipment. Pool maintenance is recommended for teens who are comfortable around the water.

5. **Data entry.** This type of work might not be suited for teens with weak motor skills or hyperactivity issues. However, those who are good with computers, and prefer working alone might enjoy this job. Community

organizations often have mailing lists that have to be maintained. And even if it is a volunteer experience, it is still good for a résumé and can result in better job opportunities in the future.

References

1. "Accommodation and Compliance: Learning Disability," Job Accommodation Network (JAN), September 19, 2011.
2. Rosen, Peg. "9 Great First-Time Jobs for Teens," Understood.org, August 31, 2014.
3. Hutchinson, Nancy L. "Literacy, Employment and Youth with Learning Disabilities," ERIC Digest, September 15, 2010.

CHAPTER 52
EMPLOYMENT SUPPORTS

About This Chapter: This chapter includes text excerpted from "Resources to Assist You Return to Work," U.S. Social Security Administration (SSA), February 3, 2008. Reviewed July 2020.

Work Incentive Liaison

An employee in each of your local Social Security offices serves as a Work Incentive Liaison (WIL) to provide advice and information about your work incentive provisions and employee support programs to individuals with disabilities and outside organizations that serve those with disabilities.

Area Work Incentives Coordinator

Area Work Incentives Coordinators (AWIC) are experienced employment support experts who:

- Coordinate and/or conduct public outreach on work incentives in their local areas
- Provide and/or coordinate and oversee training on Social Security's employment support programs for all personnel at local Social Security offices
- Handle sensitive or high profile disability work-issue cases, if necessary
- Monitor the disability work-issue workloads in their areas

Benefits Planning Query

A Benefits Planning Query (BPQY) provides information about a beneficiary's disability cash benefits, health insurance, scheduled continuing disability reviews, representative payee, and work history, as stored in Social Security's electronic records. The BPQY is an important planning tool for a beneficiary, an AWIC, Plan to Achieve Self-Support Specialist, benefits counselor, or other person who may be developing customized services for a disability beneficiary who wants to start working or stay on the job.

The BPQYs are provided to beneficiaries, their representative payees, and their authorized representatives of record upon request. Beneficiaries can request a BPQY by contacting their local Social Security office or by calling Social Security's toll-free number, 800-772-1213 between 7 a.m. and 7 p.m., Monday through Friday. People who are deaf or hard of hearing may call toll-free TTY/TDD number, 800-325-0778 between 7 a.m. and 7 p.m., Monday through Friday.

If someone other than the beneficiary, representative payee, or appointed representative (e.g., a benefits counselor) wishes to receive a BPQY, they must submit two SSA-3288 forms (Consent for Release of Information) that have been signed by the beneficiary. One is to authorize the release of Social Security records and the other to authorize the release of Internal Revenue Service earnings records. Both releases must contain the beneficiary's Social Security number or the claim number. Copies of the *SSA-3288* are available at www.ssa.gov/online/ssa-3288.pdf.

The BPQYs are also provided with free of charge if needed by the beneficiary or Ticket to Work (TTW) providers, i.e., Work Incentives Planning and Assistance (WIPAs), Protection and Advocacy for Beneficiaries of Social Security (PABSS), or Employment Networks (ENs), to assist the beneficiary to return to work under the TTW Program.

Work Incentives Planning and Assistance Projects

Work Incentives Planning and Assistance (WIPA) projects are community-based organizations that receive grants from Social Security to provide Social Security and Supplemental Security Income (SSI) disability beneficiaries, including youth in transition, free access to work incentives planning and assistance. If you are working, or interested in working, WIPA projects can give you accurate information about Social Security work incentives and other programs. Each WIPA project has counselors called "Community Work Incentives Coordinators" (CWIC) who:

- Work with you to help you understand your benefits
- Teach you when, how, and what to report to Social Security and other providers
- Provide in-depth, individualized counseling about your benefits and the effect of work on those benefits
- Provide ongoing support and information as you transition to work

If you are one of the many Social Security Disability Insurance (SSDI) or SSI disability beneficiaries who want to work, a WIPA project can help you understand the employment supports that are available to you and enable you to make informed choices about work.

WIPA services are available in every state, the District of Columbia, and the U.S. Territories of American Samoa, Guam, the Northern Mariana Islands, Puerto Rico, and the Virgin Islands. If you want to locate the WIPA organization nearest you, please call 866-968-7842 (voice) or 866-833-2967 (toll-free TTY).

Work Incentives Seminar

Work Incentives Seminar (WISE) features information to help Social Security disability beneficiaries make the decision to reenter the workforce or to work for the first time. All WISE take place via free Internet-based webinars. The webinar format allows beneficiaries and other interested parties to learn about vital employment resources from Social Security without having to travel to another location.

Some of the webinars are designed to address a broad range of disabilities, while others target people in specific disability categories or age ranges. They may feature various employment service providers, including Social Security approved Employment Networks, State Vocational Rehabilitation Agencies, Protection and Advocacy Services, and WIPA organizations. WISE topics may include Choosing a Ticket to Work Service Provider, Understanding Work Incentives and more.

Beneficiaries and other interested parties may register for scheduled WISE online via website at choosework.ssa.gov or by calling the Ticket to Work Helpline at 866-968-7842 or 866-833-2967 (toll-free TTY) Monday through Friday from 8 a.m. to 8 p.m. ET.

Employment Network and State Vocational Rehabilitation Providers

Employment Networks and State Vocational Rehabilitation agencies furnish a wide variety of services to help people with disabilities return to work, enter a new line of work, or work for the first time. You can find a list of state Employment Networks and Vocational Rehabilitation agencies in the service provider directory on the searchable tool website (*Find Help*) at choosework.ssa.gov/findhelp.

Protection and Advocacy for Beneficiaries of Social Security

In every State, U.S. Territory and the Hopi and Navajo Tribal Nations, there is an agency that protects the rights of persons with disabilities. This Protection and Advocacy for Beneficiaries of Social Security's (PABSS) system administers PABSS program. Each PABSS agency:

- Works to identify and remove barriers to employment
- Investigates any complaint you have against an employment network or other service provider that is helping you to return to work
- Gives you information and advice about vocational rehabilitation and employment services
- Tells you about Social Security's work incentives that will help you to return to work
- Provides consultation and legal representation to protect your rights in the effort to secure or regain employment
- Helps you understand and protect your employment rights, responsibilities, and reasonable accommodations under the Americans with Disabilities Act

These services are free to you if you receive SSDI or SSI benefits based on disability or blindness. If you want to locate the PABSS agency nearest you, please call 866-968-7842 (voice) or 866-833-2967 (toll-free TTY). You can also find contact information in the service provider directory at choosework.ssa.gov/findhelp.

Individual Development Accounts

If you are working and have limited income, you may be eligible for an Individual Development Accounts (IDAs) through the Temporary Assistance to Needy Families (TANF) program or an Assets for Independence Act (AFIA) grant. An IDA is a trust-like bank account that helps you save your earnings to go to school, buy a home, or start a business. When you make a deposit to the account, a participating nonprofit organization matches your deposit. The typical match is one dollar for each dollar that you deposit. The federal government adds an additional match, limited to $2,000 for an individual or $4,000 for a household over the life of the program (usually five years).

If you have an IDA through TANF or an AFIA grant, the earnings are not counted which you deposit into your account, any matching deposits, or any interest earned as SSI income or resources. As a result, your SSI benefits may increase.

Achieving a Better Life Experience

An Achieving a Better Life Experience (ABLE) account is a type of tax-advantaged account that can be used to save funds for the disability-related expenses of the account's designated beneficiary, who must be blind or disabled by a condition that began prior to her or his 26th birthday. The designated beneficiary must be:

- Receiving SSI based on disability or blindness that began before age 26
- Entitled to SSDI, Childhood Disability Benefits (CDB), or Disabled Widows or Widowers Benefits (DWB) based on disability or blindness that began before age 26
- Someone whose primary care physician has certified that she or he is disabled or blind by a condition that began before age 26

Certain qualified disability expenses can be distributed from the ABLE account if they are expenses related to the blindness or disability of the designated beneficiary. Examples of qualified disability expenses include education, housing, transportation, employment training and support, and assistive technology and related services.

American Job Centers

American Job Centers (formerly known as "One-Stop Career Centers") provide job seekers, with and without disabilities, a variety of tools and services to help them get back to work. Services include training, referrals, career counseling, job listings and other similar employment-related services. Tools, many of which are available online, assist job seekers with career exploration, skill assessments (including identifying transferable skills), credential listings, and job openings. Customers can visit a Center in person or connect to the Center's information through PC or kiosk remote access. Many American Job Centers are also Employment Networks and can accept your ticket under the Ticket to Work Program.

Job Accommodation Network

Job Accommodation Network (JAN) provides free, expert, and confidential guidance on workplace accommodations and disability employment issues to help people with disabilities enhance their employability. JAN consultants offer one-on-one guidance on workplace accommodations, the Americans with Disabilities Act and related legislation, and self-employment options for people with disabilities. Assistance is available both over the phone and online. You can contact JAN by phone at 800-526-7234 (voice) or 877-781-9403 (toll-free TTY). The JAN website (www.AskJAN.org) is a rich source of information that makes a chat service available and features the Searchable Online Accommodation Resource.

The Guidepost to Success

The Guidepost to Success is built upon extensive literature review of research, demonstration projects, and effective practices; including lessons from youth development, quality education, and workforce development programs and suggests what all youth need in order to successfully transition to adulthood. The Guideposts can help steer families, institutions, and youth themselves through the transition processes.

Financial Literacy Information for Young People with Disabilities

The financial literacy document was created based on research which shows that low educational attainment, employment expectations, and confusing governmental programs with conflicting eligibility criteria have resulted in many young people with disabilities not making successful transitions from school to postsecondary education, employment and independent living. While many would like to learn how to save money and build assets, they fear getting a job and saving a portion of their income may cause them to lose their disability benefits and other supports, such as healthcare. Complex rules in current federal and state programs often create disincentives for these youth to seek employment or increase earnings and assets. One major obstacle that contributes to this issue is the lack of money management knowledge and skills or financial literacy among this group.

Federal Employment of People with Disabilities

The federal government's Office of Personnel Management (OPM) has a special hiring authority for hiring workers that have certain significant physical, psychiatric, or mental disabilities known as "targeted disabilities."

AmeriCorps

AmeriCorps is a national network of service programs that engage Americans to meet the nation's needs in priority areas like disaster services, economic opportunity, education, environmental stewardship, healthy futures, and veterans and military families. The stipend will be excluded that AmeriCorps members receive in the determination of SSI benefits. For SSDI recipients, the income exclusion only applies to the AmeriCorps VISTA program.

CHAPTER 53

VOLUNTEERISM AND SERVICE-LEARNING AS A PATHWAY TO EMPLOYMENT

About This Chapter: This chapter includes text excerpted from "Pathway to Employment for Youth with Disabilities," Corporation for National and Community Service (CNCS), June 15, 2013. Reviewed July 2020.

Throughout the year, the Corporation for National and Community Service (CNCS) improves employment outcomes for people with disabilities, including the nation's youth with disabilities. Volunteerism can provide a great opportunity for youth with disabilities to gain important work-based skills and develop a network of contacts. Because of the untapped potential that service-learning represents, the U.S. Department of Labor's (DOL) Office of Disability Employment Policy (ODEP) and the CNCS are joining together to tell you about the importance of work-based and service-learning for all youth, including those with disabilities. In addition, the CNCS discusses income exclusions available to Social Security beneficiaries participating in service-learning opportunities under AmeriCorps, in which participants receive a living stipend.

Work-Based Learning Experiences—Why They Are Important
Work experiences, both paid and voluntary, have been recognized as critical components of preparing youth, including those with disabilities, for the transition to adulthood. In fact, the ODEP and the National Collaborative on Workforce & Disability for Youth (NCWD/Youth) cited these experiences in the Guideposts for Success. Volunteerism and service-learning are included among these on-the-job training experiences that can help prepare youth by:
- Developing career readiness skills, including basic work skills (often referred to as "soft skills"), such as attendance, punctuality, teamwork, and conflict resolution
- Providing knowledge of specific occupational skills

- Offering opportunities to establish a work history and connections
- Providing a forum for exploring different occupations

Even short-term work experiences can be valuable as a way for all youth to develop skills, contacts, and awareness about career options. Research shows that having a competitive paid job in secondary school is the strongest predictor of job success for youth with disabilities after graduation. Moreover, both paid and unpaid work experiences help youth with disabilities acquire jobs at higher wages after they graduate.

Benefits Associated with Service-Learning and Volunteerism

Numerous studies have identified that youth who participate in quality community-based service-learning experiences can gain the following benefits and others which contribute to improved transition outcomes and positive youth development:

- Access to the range of supports and opportunities (or developmental assets) they need to grow up healthy, caring, and responsible
- Increased civic engagement and community involvement
- Improved understanding of how they can impact social challenges
- Higher academic achievement and interest in furthering their education
- Enhanced problem-solving skills, ability to work in teams, and planning abilities

For youth with disabilities, service-learning provides an additional benefit. By being actively engaged in service to their communities, they gain a sense of increased self-worth associated with being providers rather than service recipients.

The Link between Volunteerism and Competitive Employment

The CNCS is an independent federal agency with the responsibility to mobilize Americans into service through three programs: Senior Corps, AmeriCorps, and The Social Innovation Fund. These programs support service-learning in schools, higher education institutions, community-based organizations, and full-time service across the nation.

New research released by CNCS in June 2013 provides the most compelling empirical research to date establishing an association between volunteering and employment in the United States. Key findings on the connection between volunteering and employment include the following:

- Volunteers have a 27 percent higher likelihood of finding a job after being out of work than nonvolunteers
- Volunteers without a high school diploma have a 51 percent higher likelihood of finding employment

- Volunteers living in rural areas have a 55 percent higher likelihood of finding employment

The CNCS also found that volunteering is associated with an increased likelihood of finding employment for all volunteers regardless of a person's gender, age, ethnicity, geographical area, or the job market conditions.

According to CNCS, volunteering can help people find employment because:
- Volunteering increases an individual's networks and connections
- Volunteering increases an individual's experience or useful education, skills, and training
- Volunteering helps to create a positive impression in a competitive job market

Income Exclusions for Service-Learning Stipends Available to Social Security Beneficiaries Participating in AmeriCorps

Despite the many benefits associated with service-learning, many youth with disabilities who are Social Security benefit recipients and their families may be hesitant to participate in such programs because they fear that they will lose these benefits. However, there are a number of income exemptions available to beneficiaries who participate in AmeriCorps.

What Is AmeriCorps?

Launched in 1993 under the National and Community Service Trust Act, AmeriCorps is a network of service programs that engage Americans to meet the nation's needs in education, public safety, health, and the environment. AmeriCorps members serve at more than 3,000 not-for-profit organizations through three programs:

Through AmeriCorps State and National, the broadest of the programs, grants are provided to a network of local and national organizations and agencies committed to using national service to address critical community needs in education, public safety, health, and the environment. AmeriCorps VISTA provides full-time members to nonprofit, faith-based and other community organizations, and public agencies to create and expand programs that bring low-income individuals and communities out of poverty. AmeriCorps National Civilian Community Corps (NCCC) is a full-time, team-based, residential program for men and women ages 18-24. Its mission is to strengthen communities and develop leaders through direct, team-based national and community service.

Currently, CNCS does not track the disability status of its service members or alumni, but volunteerism can provide an important step on the pathway to employment for youth with disabilities. AmeriCorps members receive a modest living allowance ($10,000–$14,000 for 10–12 months of service) and assistance with college costs and student loans. Some programs also provide housing.

Table 53.1. Income Exclusions for SSI and SSDI Recipients

Social Security Income Exclusions Available for AmeriCorps Programs		
	Work Incentive Available for	
	SSI Beneficiaries	SSDI Beneficiaries
AmeriCorps NCCC	X	
AmeriCorps State and Local	X	
AmeriCorps VISTA	X	X

What Income Exclusions Are Available?

Under the Heroes Earning Assistance and Relief Act (HEART Act) of 1998, AmeriCorps members with disabilities who receive Supplemental Security Income (SSI) benefits due to their disability, can receive an AmeriCorps stipend without risk of losing their disability benefits. Those participating in AmeriCorps VISTA can also receive their stipend without losing benefits related to their disability. For SSI beneficiaries, this income exclusion also includes stipends received while participating in the AmeriCorps NCCC and AmeriCorps State and Local programs.

The table above explains which AmeriCorps programs have income exclusions for SSI and SSDI recipients.

Youth, with and without disabilities, glean important benefits by engaging in work-based learning including service-learning. Moreover, although CNCS' recent research did not specifically look at volunteers with disabilities, the study suggests that volunteering is associated with an increased likelihood of finding employment particularly for volunteers who experience significant barriers when entering the workforce.

CHAPTER 54
CULTIVATING QUALIFIED WORKERS

About This Chapter: This chapter includes text excerpted from "Employment Disability 101: Lesson Two," U.S. Department of Education (ED), August 21, 2006. Reviewed July 2020.

The Next Generation of Qualified Workers

Successful companies know that meeting the growing need for talented employees in the next 10 years means educating students with the right skills now. Educators play an important role in connecting people with disabilities to employers. The Office of Special Education and Rehabilitative Services' (OSERS) Office of Special Education Programs (OSEP) works with OSERS' Rehabilitation Services Administration (RSA) and with state education agencies to prepare students with disabilities for higher education, employment, and independent living.

The OSEP also requires schools across the country to establish transition curricula, which include community work-based learning experiences for youths with disabilities. By partnering with schools to offer work-based learning experiences for students with disabilities, your business can help create a pipeline of future employees who are knowledgeable and trained for jobs in your organization. These work-based learning opportunities may include the following:

- **Apprenticeships.** On-the-job training and related classroom instruction provides students with disabilities an opportunity to learn the practical and theoretical aspects of highly skilled occupations. Joint employer and labor groups, individual employers and employer associations sponsor apprenticeship programs.
- **Career academies.** Schools create a personalized and supportive learning environment for students with disabilities by combining academic and career-related competencies organized into small learning communities.
- **Internships.** While spending time in a business, industry, or other organization, students with disabilities gain insight into and direct

experience with different types of work environments. Internships can be paid or unpaid.

- **Job shadowing and mentoring days.** These activities are designed to allow students with disabilities to "shadow" or observe workplace mentors as they go through a normal day on the job. Job shadowing and mentoring provide students with disabilities a realistic look at the workplace.
- **School-based enterprises.** Tapping into entrepreneurial talents, students with disabilities organize into a group to produce goods or services for sale. Your success as a business leader places you in a position to offer advice to these future entrepreneurs.
- **Service learning.** Students with disabilities expand their horizons by combining meaningful community service with academic learning, personal growth, and civic responsibility.

Work-based learning experiences can help students with disabilities prepare to enter your workforce and:

- Develop positive work attitudes and behaviors
- Learn general workplace readiness skills as well as job-specific skills
- Identify necessary work accommodations and supports
- Gain exposure to diverse working environments
- Apply practical theories learned in the classroom to your business
- Clarify and get excited about their career choices
- Network with potential employers

No Child Left Behind (NCLB) and the Individuals with Disabilities Education Act (IDEA) work together to give students with disabilities the educational foundation they need to be productive employees. This preparation is making a difference for our young people. The National Longitudinal Transition Study-2 (NLTS2), funded by the U.S. Department of Education (ED), shows that in 2003, 70 percent of students with disabilities who had been out of school for up to two years had paying jobs, compared to only 55 percent in 1987.

Work-Based Learning: A Win-Win Experience

Employers benefit from work-based learning experiences as well. Companies that institute mentoring, job shadowing, apprenticeship, and internship programs learn firsthand how people with disabilities can contribute. Businesses discover that working and interacting with employees with disabilities raises morale and eliminates the mystery of workplace accommodations. Positive experiences with students dispel the fears that employers have about giving people with disabilities a chance in full-time employment. Most importantly, businesses that implement these programs cultivate their next generation of qualified workers and attract new customers.

Work-Based Learning Opportunities Strategies

The strategies listed below are some of the ways you as an employer can get involved in creating work-based learning opportunities for people with disabilities in your community.

Strategy 1

Connect with your local schools by:

- Helping schools and career counselors identify competencies, both personal and technical, that students with disabilities will need in the workplace
- Instituting mentoring and internship opportunities to place students in your company-sponsored programs
- Using your business connections to provide schools with instructors in specific professional and technical fields who can work with special education and VR professionals in your community
- Assisting schools and special education coordinators to develop curricula and instructional plans that prepare students with disabilities for jobs in the local market
- Providing assistance to students who want to pursue entrepreneurial endeavors; and advising educators and counselors of the future skill needs of your workforce

To assist you in completing this strategy, locate local high schools in your area by contacting your state education agency through the Education Resource Organizations Directory (EROD) at wdcrobcolp01.ed.gov/Programs/EROD.

Strategy 2

Connect with your local community colleges and universities.

When you recruit at colleges and universities, indicate to the career office that you have an interest in recruiting students with disabilities. To provide work-based learning experiences to college students with disabilities, reach out to colleges or universities.

Strategy 3

When you attend school-sponsored open houses and job fairs, provide recruiting materials in accessible formats, make sure interviewing locations are accessible, and be sure your website is accessible to people with disabilities.

Strategy 4

Serve as a mentor to students with disabilities. Contact your local CIL (www.ilusa.com/links/ilcenters.htm) to identify possible opportunities or contact the American Association of People with Disabilities (www.aapd-dc.org) to find out how your business can participate in the annual National Disability Mentoring Day in October.

CHAPTER 55

STARTING A CAREER WITH THE FEDERAL GOVERNMENT

About This Chapter: This chapter includes text excerpted from "Federal Schedule a Hiring Authority Fact Sheet: Tips for Youth and Young Adults with Disabilities Interested in Starting a Career with the Federal Government," Youth.gov, March 15, 2012. Reviewed July 2020.

The Schedule A hiring authority (Schedule A) is one of the paths that can greatly benefit youth and young adults with disabilities who have an interest in a career with the federal government. It can also be a fast track way for federal agencies to bring in talented individuals with disabilities. When properly implemented, it is a win-win situation for both you and the hiring federal agency!

What Is Schedule A?

Schedule A is a hiring authority for federal agencies to use to tap into a diverse and vibrant talent pool without going through the often-lengthy traditional hiring process. Schedule A allows individuals to apply for a federal appointment through a non-competitive hiring process. This means that if you meet the eligibility status of the appointment and the minimum qualifications for a position, you may be hired for the position without competing with the general public. Schedule A can be used to hire people in all professions from clerical staff to attorneys.

Who Can Use Schedule A?

If you have documentation to show your disability status, you may choose to apply for federal appointments through Schedule A. People with disabilities may apply for federal appointments either using Schedule A or the traditional competitive hiring process.

Who Is Considered to Be an Individual with a Disability Status?

A youth or young adult who:

- Received Supplemental Security Income (SSI) benefits
- Identified as needing services through the Individuals with Disabilities Education Act (IDEA)
- Received services in elementary or high school through an Individualized Education Program (IEP) or a 504 plan in school
- Used Disabled Student Services on your college campus
- Needed a special accommodation
- Received vocational rehabilitation services
- Fits under the Americans with Disabilities Act's (ADA) definition of an individual with a disability

How Can Youth Document That They Are Schedule Eligible?
Introduction to Federal Government Employment
Considering a Career in Federal Government

The federal government needs leaders who bring with them a unique perspective and are determined to contribute their strengths to improve and enhance its work. Federal employees are able to make a difference through public service, receive medical benefits, and develop unique skill sets. Here are some other advantages to working for the federal government:

- Federal employees play an important role in addressing challenging and pressing national issues
- Federal salaries and benefits are competitive with the private sector
- Federal employees are given an opportunity to receive cutting-edge training and professional development to advance in the field
- The federal government may help employees pursue a graduate degree and/or help them pay back a school loan
- Most federal government agencies have policies and programs to improve life in the workplace and to assist employees in balancing their work with life responsibilities (e.g., on-site childcare, dependent care, work schedule flexibilities) regardless of academic degree, interest, or even location.

There is an opportunity for all who are interested to find a job in the federal government.

How to Find a Job in the Federal Government

The federal government's official website for job information is USAJOBS (www.usajobs.gov). Through this website, you can search for openings in a particular field, city, or agency, or all three. You also can sign up for e-mail alerts about job openings by type of job, agency, and/or geographic area. If you cannot access the Internet or need additional assistance, you can call 202-606-2525 or 978-461-8404 (TTY).

There are some federal agencies that have their own hiring system and evaluation criteria. These agencies are called "excepted service agencies." Excepted service positions, like Schedule A appointments, are not required to be posted on the USAJOBS website. As a result, it is important to look at individual agency websites for job announcements. And of course, when it comes to finding a job, networking is essential by talking with friends, family members, teachers, mentors, and acquaintances about your employment goals, interests, and desires.

How to Apply for a Federal Government Position

Those interested in applying for a federal position using Schedule A must follow the previous steps listed under Learning About Schedule A, and then contact the Hiring Manager, Human Resource (HR) professional, Disability Program Manager (DPM), and/or Selective Placement Coordinator (SPC) within the selected agency. The appropriate person or office can be found by either using the contact information included in the vacancy announcement itself (all announcements include a phone number and/or e-mail address to be used for questions) or by searching a directory of SPCs maintained by the Office of Personnel Management (OPM).

Applications should be submitted through both the regular job-posting announcement on the USAJOBS website and the individual agency website to ensure that the application is not overlooked.

CHAPTER 56

FINDING, ACCOMMODATING, AND RETAINING EMPLOYEES WITH DISABILITIES

About This Chapter: This chapter includes text excerpted from "Disability Employment 101: Lesson Three," U.S. Department of Education (ED), November 29, 2007. Reviewed July 2020.

Learning from Other Businesses

By connecting to business organizations, such as the U.S. Chamber's Center for Workforce Preparation (CWP), the U.S. Business Leadership Network, the Society for Human Resource Management and your local chamber, your company can learn from other employers about the best strategies for finding, accommodating, and retaining employees with disabilities. Local business executives who understand your bottom-line priorities and who have direct employment experience with people with disabilities are often the best sources for real-world answers to all your hiring questions.

The U.S. Chamber of Commerce's Center for Workforce Preparation

In 1990, the Chamber of Commerce created the Center for Workforce Preparation to help build workforce development leadership in local chambers. CWP helps chambers across the country to develop innovative and effective workforce development initiatives that assist their member companies in recruiting diverse and underutilized labor sources such as people with disabilities. A major part of CWP's effort is the dissemination of best practices and the formulation of strategic peer networks to support workforce development activities among state and local chambers. By connecting to CWP, you can learn how to partner with your local chamber to help improve employment outcomes for people with disabilities and to satisfy your company's workforce needs.

The U.S. Business Leadership Network

The U.S. Business Leadership Network (USBLN) is the only national employer-led organization that provides a corporate perspective to businesses regarding hiring people with disabilities and marketing to customers with disabilities. With chapters in 31 states and the District of Columbia, the USBLN is the nationally recognized disability voice for the business community because it makes the inclusion of people with disabilities a business imperative. A nonprofit trade association, the USBLN provides best practices strategies, specific industry perspectives, toolkits, and resources to employers and its 43 BLN chapters seeking to diversify their workforces by including people with disabilities.

The Society for Human Resource Management

The Society for Human Resource Management (SHRM) is the world's largest association devoted to human resource management. Representing more than 200,000 individual members, the society's mission is to serve the needs of human resource professionals by providing the most essential and comprehensive resources available, including surveys of members on disability-related topics. As an influential voice, the society's mission is also to advance the human resource profession to ensure that human resources is recognized as an essential partner in developing and executing organizational strategy. Founded in 1948, SHRM has more than 550 affiliated chapters and members in more than 100 countries.

Strategies

Strategy 1

Become a member of a USBLN chapter to network with other disability-friendly employers who are actively engaged in outreach, employment, retention, and marketing efforts to individuals with disabilities.

Strategy 2

Connect with your local chamber for information and resources about:
- Job skill requirements and industry trends
- Quality of training and job placement services provided by your local Vocational Rehabilitation program and other service providers
- Local economic development indicators
- Links to other members who have partners with local disability organizations.

Strategy 3

Access information and linkages about workforce development at CWP's website by visiting www.uschamber.com/cwp.

Strategy 4

Learn about available training that will help staff with the recruiting, hiring, and advancement of people with disabilities. One source of information is SHRM's website at www.shrm.org.

PART 7 | LIVING WITH A LEARNING DISABILITY

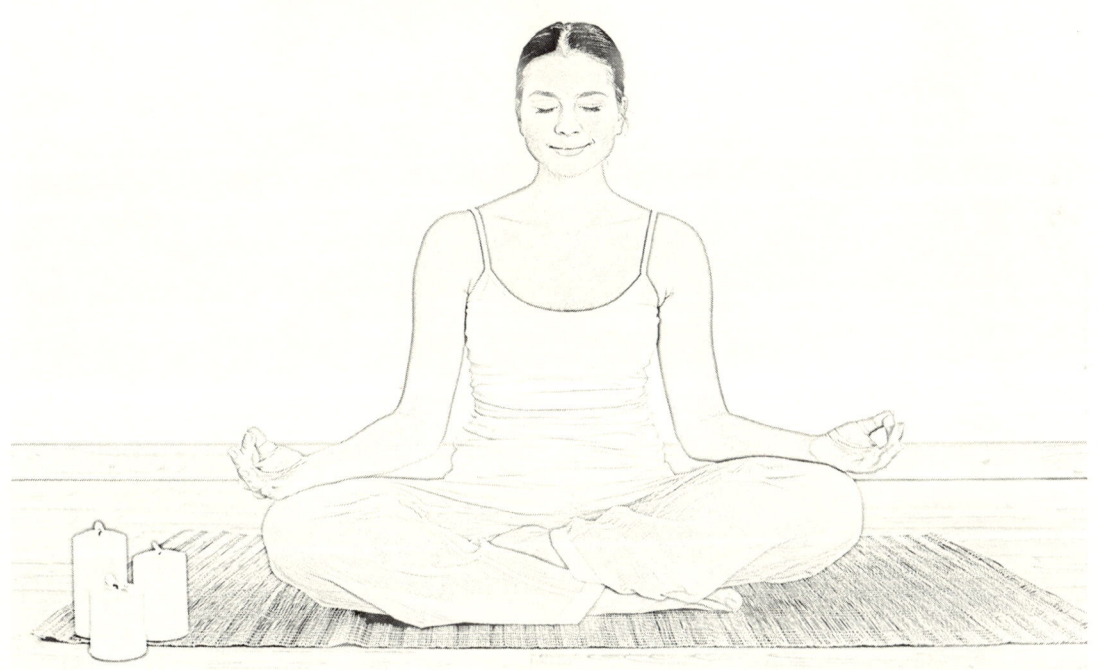

CHAPTER 57
DEEPER LEARNING

About This Chapter: "Deeper Learning," © 2020 Omnigraphics. Reviewed July 2020.

According to the National Research Council (NRC) panel, deeper learning is defined as a process that enables a person to apply what they have learned in new situations. Most schools have started including educational methods that deliver challenging academic standards using innovative techniques to master deeper learning. Deeper learning provides students with a set of skills that are required for them to succeed in both college and career. The specific definition of deeper learning varies among institutions and organizations. Still, several descriptions of deeper learning competencies include common abilities that enable a student to:

- Understand and be proficient in core academic content
- Solve complex problems using critical thinking
- Work as a team
- Incorporate criticisms
- Create an academic mindset required for learning

Deeper Learning for Students with Learning Disability

The foundation skills in reading, writing, and math are critical for deeper learning since they can be applied in various other academic domains. This can be really hard for students with learning disabilities (LDs) since they have trouble with basic comprehension, reading, or math. Due to such challenges, students with LD need to put in double the effort to learn deeper learning skills. The following are some of the practices that are known to be effective for students with considerable learning difficulties to access deeper learning:

Cognitive Processing Support

Most students with LD have trouble with cognitive processing such as memory and attention. One effective strategy for overcoming this difficulty is to teach students to define certain learning goals and self-monitor their progress. For instance, keeping a track of the number of math problems solved.

Providing Instructions

Along with instructional practices that help students with LD to understand what they are learning, more intensive support should be provided to students who require it. This involves providing instructions to those students in specific ways that are:

- **Explicit.** Clearly defined steps needed to finish a task or learn a skill.
- **Systematic.** Organizing the instructions into manageable pieces.
- **Responsive.** Receiving feedback from students on how to improve providing better instructions.

The amount of time needed to focus on a student also plays a major role in providing proper instructions, depending on the student's capacity for attention. Schools can find it quite expensive to offer deeper learning for students with disabilities since they have to hire or train teachers to provide specific instructional practices. This can also require a reduction in the size of the class and specialized services such as learning materials designed for students with LD.

Deeper Learning Assessments

There are certain strategies used to measure the knowledge and skills acquired to determine if the student has attained deeper learning. These are some of the assessment techniques used for deeper learning:

- **Performance assessment.** Applying the knowledge and skills of a student in developing a presentation or demonstration.
- **Competency assessment.** Measures specific skills of the student against a set of standards. This is done at a personalized space so it is based on how the student has mastered the content rather than the number of days it took.
- **Project-based assessment.** Observe how students apply the knowledge to a certain topic or problem over a length of time.
- **Portfolio assessment.** Collecting the students' work samples, test results, and observation records to evaluate their growth and achievement over time.

References

1. "Deeper Learning for Students with Disabilities," Students at the Center, February 15, 2015.
2. "Deepening Your Understanding of Deeper Learning," Alliance for Excellent Education, May 21, 2017.
3. "Deeper Learning," Alliance for Excellent Education, September 22, 2017.

CHAPTER 58
SERVICE-LEARNING

About This Chapter: This chapter includes text excerpted from "Service-Learning," Youth.gov, November 28, 2017.

Service-learning is a teaching and learning strategy that connects academic curriculum to community problem-solving. Nowadays, elementary, middle, high, and postsecondary schools across the nation participate in service-learning with the support of federal, state, district, and foundation funding. Studies show that, in the past, more than four million students from more than 20,000 schools participated in service-learning. Of these participants, high schools were most likely to engage students in community service or to include service-learning as part of their curriculum.

Service-learning is beneficial for students, organizations, and communities. All students, including those with disabilities (e.g., emotional and behavioral disorders, learning disabilities, moderate and severe intellectual disabilities, students with hearing and vision limitations), can be involved in and benefit from service-learning.

What Is Service-Learning?

The term "service-learning" was defined in Federal legislation for the first time in the National and Community Service Act of 1990 (as amended through December 17, 1999, P.L. 106-170; Section 101 (23) and reauthorized through Edward M. Kennedy Serve America Act of 2009):

The term "service-learning" means a method under which students or participants learn and develop through active participation in thoughtfully organized service that:

- Is conducted in and meets the needs of a community
- Is coordinated with an elementary school, secondary school, institution of higher education, or community service program, and with the community
- Helps foster civic responsibility
- That is integrated into and enhances the academic curriculum of the students, or the educational components of the community service program in which the participants are enrolled

- Provides structured time for the students or participants to reflect on the service experience

The Serve America Act of 2009 extends the purpose of service-learning to "expand and strengthen service-learning programs through year-round opportunities, including opportunities during the summer months, to improve the education of children and youth and to maximize the benefits of national and community service, in order to renew the ethic of civic responsibility and the spirit of community for children and youth throughout the United States."

The U.S. Department of Education (ED) further emphasized the importance of civic engagement and the role that schools play through service-learning and other related efforts. The Department notes that "every student in every school, college, and university deserves a high-quality education, including a high-quality civic education" in its 2012 Advancing Civic Learning and Engagement in Democracy: A Road Map and Call to Action (www.ed.gov/sites/default/files/road-map-call-to-action.pdf). The Road Map and Call to Action highlight the following five priorities:

- Advancing civic learning and democratic engagement in both the United States and global contexts by encouraging efforts to make them core expectations for elementary, secondary, and postsecondary students—including undergraduate and graduate students
- Developing more robust evidence of civic and other student achievement outcomes of civic learning, and of the impact of school and campus community partnerships
- Strengthening school and campus community connections to address significant community problems and advance a local or regional vision and narrative for civic engagement
- Expanding research and the range of public scholarship, with a special emphasis on promoting knowledge creation for the good of society
- Deepening civic identity by sharing stories of civic work in social media and organizing deliberative discussions about the roles of higher education in communities across the country, and by creating initiatives in science, arts, and other fields to catalyze civic agency

Rates

Studies show that, in the past, more than four million students from more than 20,000 schools participated in service-learning. Of these, high schools were most likely to engage students in community service or to include service-learning as part of their curriculum. All students, including those with disabilities (e.g., emotional and behavioral disorders, learning disabilities, moderate and severe intellectual disabilities, deaf and blind students), can be involved in and benefit from service-learning.

Traditionally, the number of schools that engaged students in community service was greater than the number of schools that offered service-learning as part of their curriculum. Consistently, about two-thirds of the public schools in the United States recognized or arranged community service, while only one-third of the schools offered service-learning. Service-learning is distinct from community service and volunteering because it focuses on meeting both the needs of the community and that of the learner through a mutually beneficial partnership. In addition, service-learning is integrated into academic curriculum and coursework as "a form of experiential learning which tests students' higher order thinking skills while deepening their understanding of the subject matter, their community, and themselves." It also aims to enhance civic engagement by incorporating instruction on social issues that extend beyond the immediate needs of individuals or projects.

Benefits, Challenges, and Solutions

Benefits

All youth, including those with disabilities, can benefit from participation in service-learning.

Service-Learning Can Improve Character Values and Responsible Behavior

Students can generalize what they learn from their experiences with service-learning. They learn how to be respectful toward others and toward public property, and they develop awareness of healthy life choices. Finally, they learn about cultural diversity and show more tolerance of ethnic diversity.

Service-Learning Can Improve Academic Outcomes for Students

Students participating in high-quality service-learning experiences that are meaningful (including interaction with the community, valued service activities, and relevance to students), provide time for reflection, and last for an extended period of time have been shown to make academic gains, including gains on standardized tests. In addition, students have shown increased attachment to school, engagement, and motivation. With a sample that included students with mild disabilities, researchers found similar results for academic improvement and attendance.

Service-Learning Can Promote a Sense of Connectedness to the School and the Community

A sense of connectedness includes:
- Feeling valued by community members
- Feeling responsible for the welfare of the community
- Having pride in one's community
- A high tendency to take action for the benefit of the community

Table 58.1. Challenges and Solutions of Service-learning

Challenges	Solutions
When students have negative ideas regarding service-learning that may result from community service being mandatory or negative past experience with community service, they are less likely to engage in adequate service and in self-reflection and learning associated with community service.	Address students' attitudes and expectations early in the process. Try to match sites with students' preferences and personal style. For example, students who care about interpersonal interaction may become frustrated in sites where they can have little communication with individuals. Try to clarify for students what to expect when reaching sites (e.g., the extent to which site staff will make them feel welcome).
Students may get into trouble on-sites because of behavior that may be perceived as inappropriate by individuals at the site.	Practice appropriate behavior with the students early on in the program. For example, demonstrate how to interact with elderly residents or very young children. Set a good example by maintaining a positive mood and using positive and respectful language. Know in advance the rules and expectations of the service sites, convey those rules to students, and follow up to ensure that they follow rules (e.g., avoiding disrespectful clothing and inappropriate language at a site).
Students cannot articulate the meaning of their service-learning activities. Students may not know or may not be able to articulate the purpose of participating in service-learning.	Ensure sufficient duration and intensity of the service-learning program, which will enable age-appropriate and topic-appropriate pacing of several aspects of the service-learning program, including: • Researching the topic • Preparing for community service • Putting together an action plan • Training students • Reflecting at each step of the service-learning process • Generating conclusions • Acknowledging accomplishments
Teachers may feel overburdened and resist the demands associated with service-learning. Teachers and principals may not see the value of service-learning or its relevance to students' learning. They also may feel insufficiently prepared or supported in delivering service-learning.	Schools may want to involve teachers who have successfully conducted service-learning in the past or who advocate for service-learning. In addition, giving teachers the opportunity to voice their creative ideas and empowering them to structure service-learning projects may promote teacher buy-in. Collaborate with service-learning organizations to provide teachers with adequate professional development and resources, and follow up by providing easy access to technical assistance and coaching support.

Service-Learning Can Promote Social-Emotional Skills

Researchers have found a statistically significant impact of service-learning programs on multiple outcomes, including:

- Improved social skills
- Lower levels of problem and delinquent behavior
- Better cooperation skills in the classroom
- Improved psychological well-being
- A better ability to set goals and adjust behavior to reach these goals

Frey found that students with disabilities who participated in a yearlong service-learning project had lower reports of out-of-school suspension, rule noncompliance, incidents, profanity and obscenity, physical threats and intimidation, and vandalism. Researchers also found that participation in service-learning for high school students with moderate-to-severe disabilities helped improve students' sense of self-worth. Researchers also found improvements for students with moderate to profound disabilities in socialization skills and their relationships with nondisabled peers.

Service-Learning Can Promote Civic Participation

Research has shown that high-quality service-learning programs can promote students' civic knowledge and commitment to continue contributing to their community and to society as a whole.

Challenges and Solutions

Researchers have documented common school-level challenges or roadblocks associated with service-learning. Educators should consider these potential roadblocks when planning to implement a local service-learning program.

Best Practices

Policies and Practices to Support Implementation

Policies at the national, state, and district levels that support service-learning can legitimize the practice of service-learning as a key component of education. These policies can also provide resources, professional development, and guidelines for service-learning programs. They can ensure successful implementation and sustainability of school-based service-learning programs.

State-Level Policies

A 2014 scan of state policies suggests that many states are adopting policies that both support and regulate the practice of service-learning (e.g., graduation requirements, funding, implementation guidance).

Table 58.2. State-Level Policies

Policies and Guidance Related to Service-Learning	Number of States	States
Permit community service or service-learning activities to count toward high school graduation requirements	22	Arkansas; Connecticut; Delaware; Florida; Georgia; Hawaii; Illinois; Indiana; Minnesota; Missouri; Nevada; New Hampshire; New Jersey; New Mexico; North Dakota; Ohio; Oklahoma; Oregon; South Dakota; Tennessee; Texas; Washington; West Virginia
Require service-learning for high school graduation statewide	2	Maryland; District of Columbia
Permit individual districts to adopt service-learning requirement for high school graduation	6	Colorado; Florida; Iowa; Rhode Island; Tennessee; Wisconsin
Provide funding for service-learning activities and programs	11	Arkansas; California; Florida; Georgia; Illinois; Iowa; Minnesota; Missouri; New York; Washington; Wyoming
Encourage the use of service-learning as an instructional method for increasing student achievement	16	California; Colorado; Delaware; Florida; Georgia; Indiana; Iowa; Michigan; Mississippi; Missouri; New York; Ohio; Oregon; Rhode Island; Utah; West Virginia
Encourage the use of service-learning as an instructional method for increasing student civic engagement	18	Alabama; California; Delaware; District of Columbia; Florida; Illinois; Michigan; Mississippi; Missouri; Montana; New Hampshire; New Jersey; Oklahoma; Rhode Island; South Dakota; Tennessee; Utah; Virginia
Encourage the use of service-learning as an instructional method for preparing students for the workforce	23	California; Colorado; Connecticut; Florida; Georgia; Kentucky; Louisiana; Michigan; Montana; Nebraska; New Mexico; New York; North Carolina; North Dakota; Ohio; Oklahoma; Oregon; Pennsylvania; Rhode Island; South Carolina; Tennessee; Utah; West Virginia
Included service-learning as part of the state's education standards and/or frameworks	33	Alaska; California; Colorado; Delaware; Florida; Idaho; Indiana; Kentucky; Louisiana; Maine; Massachusetts; Michigan; Mississippi; Missouri; Montana; Nebraska; Nevada; New Hampshire; New Jersey; New Mexico; New York; North Dakota; Ohio; Oklahoma; Oregon; Pennsylvania; Rhode Island; South Dakota; Tennessee; Texas; Vermont; Virginia; West Virginia
Support/encourage/require service-learning professional development for teachers	13	Colorado; Connecticut; Florida; Georgia; Minnesota; Missouri; Montana; New Hampshire; New Mexico; Ohio; Oklahoma; Tennessee; Utah
Support/encourage/require service-learning professional development for administrators	1	Colorado

Table 58.2. continued

Policies and Guidance Related to Service-Learning	Number of States	States
Other guidance related to service-learning	27	Arizona; California; Colorado; Florida; Kansas; Kentucky; Louisiana; Maine; Maryland; Massachusetts; Minnesota; Nebraska; New Hampshire; New York; North Carolina; North Dakota; Ohio; Oklahoma; Oregon; Pennsylvania; Rhode Island; Tennessee; Texas; Utah; Vermont; Virginia; Wisconsin

District-Level Policies

Research shows that schools with a district policy in place are much more likely to participate in service-learning (51%) than schools without a district policy (17%) or when the policy is unknown (21%).

The majority of schools implementing service-learning integrate it into at least one aspect of school policies. Such policies may include one or more of the following:

- Integration of service-learning as a part of the board-approved course curriculum for at least one subject area in at least one grade level
- Recognition of service-learning in the school improvement plan
- Inclusion of service-learning in teacher and staff orientation
- Consideration of service-learning as a criterion for teacher and staff evaluation

Integration into Curriculum and Policies

According to the National Study of the Prevalence of Community Service and Service-Learning in K-12 public schools, for schools that have service-learning, 39 percent include service-learning in the board-approved curriculum for at least one subject in one grade level.

School principals in schools that implement service-learning reported that service-learning was most likely to take place in social studies, science, and English/language arts:

- 52 percent of principals reported that service-learning was included in core curriculum for social studies
- 42 percent of principals reported that service-learning was included in core curriculum for science
- 34 percent of principals reported that service-learning was included in core curriculum for English/language arts

While less frequent, principals also reported that service-learning was incorporated into:

- Art, music, and theater
- Career education

- Mathematics
- Health
- Special education
- Gifted/talented education
- Physical education
- Foreign languages

District policies that support service-learning can legitimize the practice of service-learning as a key component of education. These policies can also provide resources, professional development, and guidelines for service-learning programs. As such, they can ensure successful implementation and sustainability of school-based service-learning programs.

Principles and Standards of Effective Programs

The following summarizes the eight standards developed and released by the National Youth Leadership Council (NYLC) in 2008.

Service-Learning Actively Engages Participants in Meaningful and Personally Relevant Service Activities

To meet this standard, service-learning needs to be:
- Age-appropriate and personally relevant
- Interesting and engaging
- Well-understood by participants in the context of social issues addressed
- Outcome-oriented with specific attainable outcomes

Service-Learning Is Intentionally Used as an Instructional Strategy to Meet Learning Goals and/or Content Standards

To meet this standard, programs need to:
- Have clearly stated goals
- Be aligned with the academic curriculum
- Include explicit teaching of transferring skills from one setting to another
- For school-based programs, be formally recognized in school board policies and in student records

Service-Learning Incorporates Multiple Challenging Reflection Activities That Are Ongoing and That Prompt Deep Thinking and Analysis about Oneself and One's Relationship to Society

Students should participate in a variety of activities to demonstrate changes in their knowledge, skills, or attitudes. Additionally, students should examine their beliefs, assumptions, and attitudes about issues, perceptions of their roles as members of their community, and the overarching issues of community problems.

Service-Learning Promotes Understanding of Diversity and Mutual Respect among All Participants

To meet this standard, programs should integrate teaching focused on taking the perspective of the other, resolving conflicts, and promoting tolerance of diversity and overcoming stereotypes.

Service-Learning Provides Youth with a Strong Voice in Planning, Implementing, and Evaluating Service-Learning Experiences with Guidance from Adults

Service-learning programs should consistently integrate opportunities for participants to voice their opinions, propose ideas and solutions, and participate in decision-making processes.

Service-Learning Partnerships Are Collaborative, Mutually-Beneficial, and Address Community Needs

Service-learning programs should engage a variety of partners—including youth, educators, families, community members, community-based organizations, and/or businesses—in communications, knowledge sharing, and goal-setting.

Service-Learning Engages Participants in an Ongoing Process to Assess the Quality of Implementation and Progress toward Meeting Specified Goals and Uses Results for Improvement and Sustainability

Service-learning programs should encourage participants to:
- Collect evidence of progress toward specific service goals and learning outcomes as well as the quality of implementation
- Use and communicate the evidence to improve the service-learning experience

Service-Learning Has Sufficient Duration and Intensity to Address Community Needs and Meet Specified Outcomes

Service-learning programs should include a needs sensing and planning time to determine the time needed for the project, be conducted during specific periods of time, and be implemented long enough to achieve the service goals and learning outcomes.

Diversity and Intercultural Service-Learning

Service-learning offers rich opportunities for students to understand and experience diversity in meaningful ways, demystifies stereotypes, and provides a way for students to learn about other cultures and to explore differences, including race, gender, ethnicity, socioeconomic status, geographic location, environment, values, beliefs, traditions, and abilities.

Importance of Intercultural Service-Learning

Given the interconnectedness of our global communities, the issues of intercultural respect and dialogue have become the highlight of national and international discussions. Because youth represent the future, their participation in successful intercultural service projects on the local, national, and international levels can have an impact on global issues that affect all of us. When service and intercultural learning are combined, young people are able to contribute their time and talent from the perspective of their own diverse backgrounds and enrich not only their own lives but also the lives of those with whom they come into contact. Cooperating with youth from other countries, cultures, regions, or communities of the world can result in dialogue, tolerance, and universal peace. Moreover, intercultural service-learning projects allow young people around the world to expose and address multifaceted local, national, and global problems. These opportunities contribute to the development of civic responsibility among youth in partnering communities throughout the world and also allow them to design sustainable efforts that focus on issues such as disaster relief, famine, equal rights, poverty, disease, and more.

CHAPTER 59
SCHOOL SUPPORTIVE LEARNING ENVIRONMENT

About This Chapter: This chapter includes text excerpted from "School Climate Improvement," U.S. Department of Education (ED), August 9, 2013. Reviewed July 2020.

School climate is a broad, multifaceted concept that involves many aspects of the student's educational experience. A positive school climate is the product of a school's attention to fostering safety; promoting a supportive academic, disciplinary, and physical environment; and encouraging and maintaining respectful, trusting, and caring relationships throughout the school community no matter the setting—from Pre-K/Elementary school to higher education.

A positive school climate is critically related to school success. For example, it can improve attendance, achievement, and retention, and even rates of graduation, according to research. School climate has many aspects. Defining a framework for understanding school climate can help educators identify key areas to focus on to create safe and supportive climates in their schools.

School Climate Describes School Conditions That Influence Student Learning (Safe Supportive School/EDSCLS Model)

According to the Safe and Supportive Schools Model, which was developed by a national panel of researchers and other experts, positive school climate involves:

- **Engagement**. Strong relationships between students, teachers, families, and schools and strong connections between schools and the broader community.
- **Safety**. Schools and school-related activities where students are safe from violence, bullying, harassment, and controlled-substance use.
- **Environment**. Appropriate facilities, well-managed classrooms, available school-based health supports, and a clear, fair disciplinary policy.

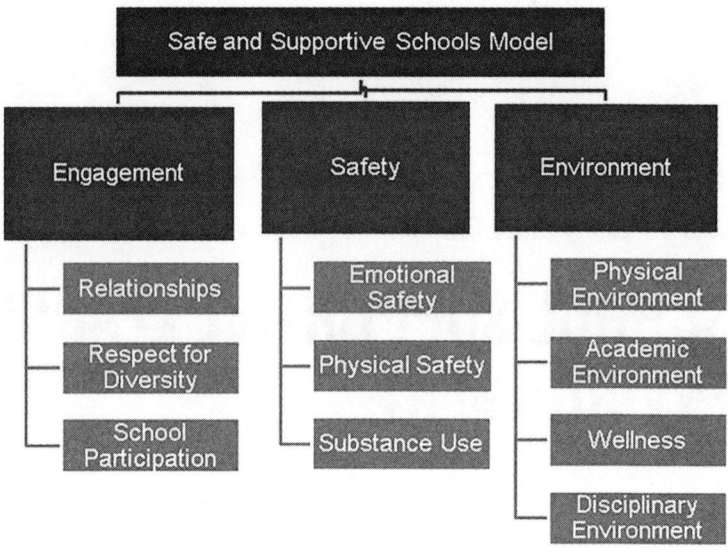

Figure 59.1. Safe and Supportive Schools Model

These areas overlap in many existing frameworks of school climate, and it is critical that all three areas be considered as a single issue in policy and practice.

School Climate Affects Student Learning

Research has shown that a positive school climate is tied to high or improving attendance rates, test scores, promotion rates, and graduation rates. For example, a 2008 study examined seven years of longitudinal data on school leadership, parent and community ties, faculty quality, school safety and order, and instructional guidance. Schools that measured strong in most supports were 10 times as likely as schools with one or two strengths to show substantial gains in reading and mathematics.

Conversely, a negative school climate can harm students and raise liability issues for schools and districts. Negative school climate is linked to lower student achievement and graduation rates, and it creates opportunities for violence, bullying, and even suicide.

The Safe and Supportive Schools Model demonstrates general consensus among researchers and practitioners on many common characteristics of schools with a positive climate. Some researchers use the concept of creating conditions for learning in speaking about school climate, meaning that students are supported, students are socially capable, students are safe, and students are challenged. Others have outlined the importance of climate at the classroom level.

The strength of the linkages between school climate and academic achievement makes it essential that all students have the opportunity to attend schools that provide a safe and supportive environment where they can thrive and fully engage in their studies.

CHAPTER 60
ASSISTIVE TECHNOLOGY

About This Chapter: Text under the heading "Built-Up Grip for Pencil or Paintbrush" is excerpted from "Built-Up Grip for Pencil or Paintbrush," National Institute on Disability, Independent Living, and Rehabilitation Research (NIDILRR), Administration for Community Living (ACL), March 8, 2006. Reviewed July 2020; Text under the heading "Right-Line Paper and Stop-Go Right-Line Paper" is excerpted from "Right-Line Paper and Stop-Go Right-Line Paper," National Institute on Disability, Independent Living, and Rehabilitation Research (NIDILRR), Administration for Community Living (ACL), May 12, 2008. Reviewed July 2020; Text under the heading "Franklin Talking Dictionary" is excerpted from "Franklin Talking Dictionary," National Institute on Disability, Independent Living, and Rehabilitation Research (NIDILRR), Administration for Community Living (ACL), December 12, 2012. Reviewed July 2020; Text under the heading "Assistive Technology Products for Information Access" is excerpted from "Assistive Technology Products for Information Access," U.S. Library of Congress (LOC), November 9, 2016. Reviewed July 2020; Text under the heading "Neo N2 Smartpen with Neo Notes App" is excerpted from "Device Review: Neo N2 Smartpen with Neo Notes App by Neo Smartpen," U.S. Department of Veterans Affairs (VA), April 23, 2018; Text under the heading "Livescribe Pulse" is excerpted from "Device Review: Livescribe Pulse by Livescribe," U.S. Department of Veterans Affairs (VA), September 9, 2010. Reviewed July 2020; Text under the heading "Auxiliary Aids and Services for Postsecondary Students with Disabilities" is excerpted from "Auxiliary Aids and Services for Postsecondary Students with Disabilities," U.S. Department of Education (ED), January 10, 2020; Text under the heading "Talking Tape Measure" is excerpted from "Talking Tape Measure," National Institute on Disability, Independent Living, and Rehabilitation Research (NIDILRR), Administration for Community Living (ACL), October 27, 2010. Reviewed July 2020; Text under the heading "Mathpad By Voice" is excerpted from "Mathpad By Voice," National Institute on Disability, Independent Living, and Rehabilitation Research (NIDILRR), Administration for Community Living (ACL), March 21, 2011. Reviewed July 2020.

Built-Up Grip for Pencil or Paintbrush

Do it yourself (DIY) Built-Up Grip Pencil or Paintbrush provide an enlarged grasping surface for individuals with arthritis or fine motor or grasping disabilities. The barrel of a pen, the shaft of a pencil, or the handle of a paintbrush can be pressed through the center of a two-inch foam ball, a Ping-Pong ball, or a hollow plastic, practice golf ball.

Right-Line Paper and Stop-Go Right-Line Paper

Right-Line and Stop-Go Right-Line paper is writing paper with raised lines designed for use by people who have difficulty staying within the lines of other writing paper such as individuals with upper extremity or fine motor disabilities or vision impairment. Both papers are printed on white stock. Right-Line paper has raised lines superimposed on printed green lines to allow the user to feel the line. Stop-Go Right-Line has red and green printed lines, with the raised line superimposed on the red lines to allow the student to see and feel the base and top lines. Right-Line is available in wide- or narrow-ruled sheets or mixed packages. (Wide-ruled paper has a dashed guideline for letter formation between the two raised lines.)

Franklin Talking Dictionary

The Franklin Talking Dictionary is a voice output dictionary designed for use by individuals who are blind or have low vision or learning disabilities. This handheld unit functions as a dictionary, thesaurus, spelling corrector, and English language resource. Every letter, word, phrase, definition, synonym, help message, menu, and game talks at various volumes and speeds. Every word can be heard letter by letter or sound by sound. Every key speaks its letter or function. The typewriter style keyboard has high contrast lettering and raised press on locator dots and a large screen with 0.25 inch display characters. It is portable and comes with cassette and print instruction manuals, headphones for private listening and carry case. POWER: Four "AA" batteries or AC adapter (both included). DIMENSIONS: 5.5 x 5 x 1 inches. WEIGHT: 11 ounces. WARRANTY: One year.

Assistive Technology Products for Information Access

The products are designed to assist people who have visual or physical disabilities in accessing printed information. They convert digital text or print into synthetic speech, braille, or enlarged text.

Neo N2 Smartpen with Neo Notes App

The Neo N2 smartpen with Neo Notes app is a slick, lightweight pen that records handwritten data and syncs electronically to Neo Notes and Evernote apps. This product has potential clinical applications for polytrauma patients with mild-to-moderate cognitive deficits who are returning to work and/or school.

Indications

Patients with mild to moderately impaired attention, memory, organization, planning and self-monitoring, secondary to medical, psychiatric and/or psychological disorders, could benefit from use of this device. Specifically, motivated patients who are actively pursuing or currently participating in work and/or school. Clinicians assessing patients should consider a full clinical profile when determining if this product is clinically indicated. Patients with documented, current (<1year), objective assessments in addition to functional need for devices to be successful in a vocational and/or scholastic setting, is necessary prior to issuing a device. Patients should have adequate fine motor abilities to write with devices and own a personal tablet or smart device (android or iOS).

Livescribe Pulse

The Livescribe Pulse smartpen is a pen that records audio while taking handwritten notes and links the notes to the audio content using a camera on the pen and a dot pattern on the special-purpose Livescribe paper. The pen's single-line LED screen offers menu feedback and a playback timeline.

The smartpen has three audio-sensitivity settings: automatic, lecture hall, and conference room. Depending on the situation users can choose the appropriate setting. The smartpen does a remarkable job of picking up sounds in even the most difficult situations. One downside is that users might pick up the scraping sound of the pen dragging on the paper; but this generally is not distracting and would not hinder the user's ability to discern who was talking or what they were saying. The standout feature of the Pulse smartpen is that it keeps the audio and your notes in sync. Placing the nib of the smartpen at any point of the notes will cause the corresponding audio to play through the pen's speaker, allowing the user to retrieve the context for her or his written notes.

The smartpen has the ability to capture 100 hours of audio (on the 2GB version). Livescribe Desktop software supports copying both the recorded audio and the visual notes to a computer. This relatively basic application manages the firmware of the pen and all the data you collect. The Livescribe Desktop software can download written notes and audio into "sessions." The software can manage multiple pens and notebooks. Selecting one of your notebooks in the Page views brings up thumbnail views of all the pages in the notebook. A double click brings the page into full view, and a zoom slider bar allows for zooming in on any part of the page. The image-capture variety is near perfect. All text starts as pale green and fills in as dark green during audio playback. You can click on any part of the written notes to hear the corresponding audio.

Every smartpen user gets 500MB of free storage at Livescribe Online. In addition to storage, there is a community where users can post pages they have written or drawn, and people can comment on their work.

Though the device was not specifically designed as assistive technology for cognition, it can be used as an external memory aid to record knowledge and improve prospective memory functioning. The smartpen has the advantage of being minimally intrusive, and facilitates the activity of note taking without requiring the intervention of another individual as a dedicated note taker. The smartpen thereby provides an opportunity for inclusion within an educational or vocational setting.

The smartpen can be utilized as an organizing system (e.g., memory log) or an external cueing system (e.g., list of instructions with audio).

The long-term successes of the individual using the device will depend on reviewing and archiving the note-taking content and developing prospective lists for each day's activities. Some users may be able to perform these activities independently, while others will need support from a personal assistant.

Indications

This device is indicated for individuals with mild cognitive disabilities, limited motor speed or even motoric abilities. However, it still allows a note taker to take notes and allows alternate computer access to manipulate the information. The key to utilizing the device is the ability to learn the process for recording and replaying handwritten text and audio. Specifically, the individuals need to learn to enter information, review information, and delete information.

Auxiliary Aids and Services for Postsecondary Students with Disabilities

Some of the various types of auxiliary aids and services may include:

- Taped texts
- Notetakers
- Interpreters
- Readers
- Videotext displays
- Television enlargers
- Talking calculators
- Electronic readers
- Braille calculators, printers, or typewriters
- Telephone handset amplifiers
- Closed caption decoders
- Open and closed captioning
- Voice synthesizers
- Specialized gym equipment
- Calculators or keyboards with large buttons
- Reaching device for library use
- Raised-line drawing kits
- Assistive listening devices
- Assistive listening systems
- Telecommunications devices for deaf persons

Technological advances in electronics have improved vastly participation by students with disabilities in educational activities. Colleges are not required to provide the most sophisticated auxiliary aids available; however, the aids provided must effectively meet the needs of a student with a disability. An institution has flexibility in choosing the specific aid or service it provides to the student, as long as the aid or service selected is effective. These aids should be selected after consultation with the student who will use them.

Effectiveness of Auxiliary Aids

No aid or service will be useful unless it is successful in equalizing the opportunity for a particular student with a disability to participate in the education program or activity. Not all students with a similar disability benefit equally from an identical auxiliary aid or service. The regulation refers to this complex issue of effectiveness in several sections, including:

- Auxiliary aids may include taped texts, interpreters or other effective methods of making orally delivered materials available to students with hearing impairments, readers in libraries for students with visual impairments, classroom equipment adapted for use by students with manual impairments, and other similar services and actions.

There are other references to effectiveness in the general provisions of the Section 504 regulation which state, in part, that a recipient may not:

- Provide a qualified handicapped person with an aid, benefit, or service that is not as effective as that provided to others
- Provide different or separate aid, benefits, or services to handicapped persons or to any class of handicapped persons unless such action is necessary to provide qualified handicapped persons with aid, benefits, or services that are as effective as those provided to others

Cost of Auxiliary Aids

Postsecondary schools receiving federal financial assistance must provide effective auxiliary aids to students who are disabled. If an aid is necessary for classroom or other appropriate (nonpersonal) use, the institution must make it available, unless provision of the aid would cause undue burden. A student with a disability may not be required to pay part or all of the costs of that aid or service. An institution may not limit what it spends for auxiliary aids or services or refuse to provide auxiliary aids because it believes that other providers of these services exist, or condition its provision of auxiliary aids on availability of funds. In many cases, an institution may meet its obligation to provide auxiliary aids by assisting the student in obtaining the aid or obtaining reimbursement for the cost of an aid from an outside agency or organization, such as a state rehabilitation agency or a private charitable organization. However, the institution remains responsible for providing the aid.

Personal Aids and Services

An issue that is often misunderstood by postsecondary officials and students is the provision of personal aids and services. Personal aids and services, including help in bathing, dressing, or other personal care, are not required to be provided by postsecondary institutions. The Section 504 regulation states:

- Recipients need not provide attendants, individually prescribed devices, readers for personal use or study, or other devices or services of a personal nature.
- Title II of the ADA similarly states that personal services are not required.

In order to ensure that students with disabilities are given a free appropriate public education, local education agencies are required to provide many services and aids of a personal nature to students with disabilities when they are enrolled in elementary and secondary schools. However, once students with disabilities graduate from a high school program or its equivalent, education institutions are no longer required to provide aids, devices, or services of a personal nature.

Postsecondary schools do not have to provide personal services relating to certain individual academic activities. Personal attendants and individually prescribed devices are the responsibility of the student who has a disability and not of the institution. For example, readers may be provided for classroom use, but institutions are not required to provide readers for personal use or for help during individual study time.

Talking Tape Measure

The Talking Tape Measure is an audible tape measure designed for use by individuals who are blind or have low vision. This tape measure features buttons to dispense and retract the tape, metric conversion buttons, and an on/off switch. At the press of a button, the measurement is announced. The unit measures up to 16 feet and automatically shuts off after the measurement is given. A belt clip and case are included.

MathPad By Voice

MathPad By Voice is a voice input version of MathPad designed for students who have upper extremity disabilities. MathPad By Voice enables students with upper extremity disabilities to do classroom arithmetic exercises and homework, including addition, subtraction, multiplication, and division, through voice input. MathPad by Voice also reads back the student's work and checks her or his answers. Work can be saved or printed. Teachers can also use MathPad By Voice to prepare homework. A print manual/tutorial is included.

- Compatilibility. For use on IBM and compatible computers.
- System Requirements. NaturallySpeaking Professional or DragonDictate; a 300 megahertz (MHz) or faster processor, 128 megabytes (MB) random access memory (RAM) for NaturallySpeaking Professional or 64 MB RAM for DragonDictate; and SoundBlaster or compatible sound card.

CHAPTER 61

SELF-ESTEEM ISSUES AND CHILDREN WITH LEARNING DISABILITIES

"Self-esteem" refers to positive feelings of worth, acceptance, and value that people hold with regard to themselves. Children who have high self-esteem feel proud, confident, secure, and capable. These feelings enable them to act independently, take responsibility for their actions, stand up for themselves, and face challenges. They are more likely to be resilient and keep trying if they make a mistake, and to have the courage to make good decisions in the face of peer pressure. Children with low self-esteem, on the other hand, lack confidence and do not believe they have value and are worthy of respect. They are less likely to stand up for themselves or ask for help, and they are more likely to give in to peer pressure.

How Self-Esteem Develops

"Self-esteem" begins to develop in infancy. In childhood, when the primary influences are loving parents, most people have very positive self-esteem. Toddlers, for instance, often respond with enthusiasm when asked if they are smart or able to do something. Young children try new things, experience repeated successes, and receive praise for their efforts. This pattern gives them confidence to face additional challenges and makes them feel good about themselves. Over time, they develop the positive characteristics associated with high self-esteem.

As children reach school age, however, they gradually begin incorporating more negative feedback from the classroom and other parts of the outside world. They experience failures, and their efforts are not always rewarded. Around the age of seven, children begin comparing themselves to their peers and realizing that others may possess stronger skills in some areas. As a result, their confidence and self-esteem may begin to wane.

Learning Disabilities and Self-Esteem

This process affects children with learning disabilities to a greater degree than most other children. Children with learning disabilities tend to experience more failure and receive more negative feedback. They also compare themselves unfavourably to their peers in terms of academic skills and performance. Schoolwork comes less easily to them and can sometimes seem impossible. Although many children with learning disabilities or attention issues are accepted by their peers, some become targets of teasing or bullying.

As a result, research suggests that children with learning disabilities tend to have lower self-esteem than their peers. After years of academic struggles and frustration, they often view themselves as being "stupid" or "slow" in comparison with other children. They tend to generalize these feelings and perceive themselves negatively in other areas of life as well. Due to low self-esteem, children with learning disabilities may lose interest in learning, develop self-defeating ways of dealing with challenges, and perform poorly, which only reinforces their low self-worth.

Ways Parents Can Impact Self-Esteem

Fortunately, parents, siblings, friends, teachers, and other influential people can help bolster children's self-esteem. Experts stress that it is possible for children to learn to improve the way they view themselves and their abilities. For parents of children with learning disabilities, being supportive yet realistic is the key to helping children build their self-esteem. While praise and positive feedback is important, it becomes meaningless if it is offered insincerely. When parents lavish praise on everything a child does, the child may begin to distrust it or overreact to negative feedback. Parents can incorporate the following suggestions to help children with learning disabilities develop higher self-esteem:

- Emphasize that the child is bright and healthy, and that they just have a deficit in a certain area of learning.
- Encourage the child's nonacademic interests—such as art, music, or sports—and highlight their areas of strength—such as kindness or a sense of humor.
- Provide an example of how to value personal strengths while also acknowledging and working to improve upon weaknesses.
- Offer examples of successful people who have overcome learning disabilities and achieved their dreams.
- Express clear, realistic expectations instead of criticisms. For instance, instead of complaining that the child's room is always messy, ask the child to put away their toys and make their bed.
- Ensure that the child has plenty of opportunities to be successful.
- Help the child view mistakes as learning experiences for next time.

- Avoid comparing the child to other people—such as siblings or classmates—and only evaluate their performance in relation to previous efforts.
- Help the child develop positive strategies for learning and coping with challenges.
- Help the child build effective problem-solving and decision-making skills. Rather than providing solutions, help them brainstorm creative approaches and consider the possible consequences of each one.
- Teach the child to reframe negative statements.
- Help the child find friends who accept them and make them feel valued.
- Encourage the child to help others by volunteering in the community. Having something valuable to offer to other people bolsters self-esteem.
- Provide a safe haven where the child feels loved, appreciated, and supported. Studies show that children who are made to feel special by an adult develop increased hopefulness and resilience.

Self-esteem is a tremendous asset to help children manage learning disabilities successfully. Parents can play an important role in building self-confidence and empowering children with learning disabilities to overcome the challenges they face.

References

1. Cunningham, Bob. "The Importance of Self-Esteem for Kids with Learning and Attention Issues," Understood.org, 2016.
2. Lyons, Aoife. "Self-Esteem and Learning Disabilities," Learning Disabilities Association (LDA) of Illinois, 2012.
3. Tracey, Danielle. "Self-Esteem and Children's Learning Problems," Learning Links, November 2012.

CHAPTER 62

SELF-ADVOCACY FOR STUDENTS WITH LEARNING DISABILITIES

About This Chapter: "Self-Advocacy for Students with Learning Disabilities," © 2017 Omnigraphics. Reviewed July 2020.

Speaking up for yourself is never easy. It is common to feel nervous or embarrassed when you have to approach a teacher to ask for extra time to complete an assignment, for instance, or tell a classmate that they are doing something that bothers you. The ability to express your feelings, ask for what you want, and promote your own interests is called "self-advocacy." It is a valuable skill to learn—especially for teens with learning disabilities. Becoming a self-advocate means playing a more active role in decisions that affect your life. Self-advocacy empowers you to take greater control over situations you face at school, at work, or in the community. For teens with learning disabilities, self-advocacy also involves understanding your rights, requesting accommodations, and accessing the services and supports you need to be successful.

How to Become a Self-Advocate

Up to now, adults may have stepped in to advocate for you in educational or social settings. As you transition to adulthood, however, you will need to take greater responsibility for protecting your own rights and interests. Luckily, it is possible to develop or strengthen self-advocacy skills. Here are some tips for learning to be an effective self-advocate:

- **Know yourself.** Before you can speak up for yourself, you need to understand what you want and need. After all, learning strategies and accommodations that work for one student may not be the best ones for you. Thinking about your strengths and weaknesses, and the tools and strategies that best complement your learning style, allows you to be specific in asking for help.

- **Know your rights.** If you have a diagnosed learning disability, you have the legal right to reasonable accommodations at school or at work. In order to self-advocate for those rights, however, you need to understand exactly what they are. Learn how disability law applies to your situation and know the details of your Individualized Education Plan (IEP). This way, you will be well-equipped to play a bigger role in your own educational decisions.

- **Practice speaking up.** Once you understand your personal needs and your rights under the law, you are ready to begin speaking up. You could start by sharing your thoughts and opinions in everyday situations. Some examples include raising your hand in class or joining a family discussion at the dinner table. Next, you could try asking questions to clarify what your teacher, counselor, or doctor says. As you begin to gain confidence, you can expand your self-advocacy to include asking for accommodations or standing up for your rights. If self-advocacy makes you feel nervous, you might find it helpful to practice what you want to say ahead of time. You could write down your main points and say them out loud to a trusted friend or to yourself in front of the mirror. Your goals should be to strike a balance between being assertive and being respectful. Other people will be more likely to listen to your concerns and try to help you if you approach them as problem-solving partners rather than adversaries.

- **Build a supportive team.** Self-advocacy becomes much easier when you have a team of supportive people on your side. People you know and trust—including friends, family members, teachers, academic advisors, doctors, counselors, coaches, and religious leaders—are usually eager to help you become a strong self-advocate. You may also gain confidence and feel more comfortable asking for accommodations by speaking with fellow students who receive support for learning disabilities. Forming a community of self-advocates can help everyone achieve their common goals.

Although self-advocacy may feel awkward or scary, it is important to remember that you have the right to ask for the resources you need to be happy and successful. You should not feel embarrassed about needing help, and you should not give up if you run into obstacles. Self-advocacy is a skill that you can learn, practice, and improve over time. Mastering it will give you the power to make choices and determine the course of your own life.

References

1. McLelland, Corrin. "Self-Advocacy," Disability Rights UK, April 20, 2015.
2. Weigel, Dessie. "Self-Advocacy: Five Tips from a Student," National Center for Learning Disabilities (NCLD), 2017.
3. "Youth in Action! Becoming a Stronger Self-Advocate," National Collaborative on Workforce and Disability for Youth (NCWD/Youth), 2015.

CHAPTER 63

COMMON BARRIERS TO PARTICIPATION EXPERIENCED BY PEOPLE WITH DISABILITIES

About This Chapter: This chapter includes text excerpted from "Disability and Health Disability Barriers," Centers for Disease Control and Prevention (CDC), September 4, 2019.

Nearly everyone faces hardships and difficulties at one time or another. But, for people with disabilities, barriers can be more frequent and have greater impact. The World Health Organization (WHO) describes barriers as being more than just physical obstacles. Here is the WHO definition of barriers:
- Factors in a person's environment that, through their absence or presence, limit functioning and create disability. These include aspects such as:
  - A physical environment that is not accessible
  - Lack of relevant assistive technology (assistive, adaptive, and rehabilitative devices)
  - Negative attitudes of people towards disability
  - Services, systems, and policies that are either nonexistent or that hinder the involvement of all people with a health condition in all areas of life

Often there are multiple barriers that can make it extremely difficult or even impossible for people with disabilities to function. Here are the seven most common barriers. Often, more than one barrier occurs at a time.
- Attitudinal
- Communication
- Physical
- Policy
- Programmatic
- Social
- Transportation

Attitudinal Barriers

Attitudinal barriers are the most basic and contribute to other barriers. For example, some people may not be aware that difficulties in getting to or into a place can limit a person with a disability from participating in everyday life and common daily activities. Examples of attitudinal barriers include:

- **Stereotyping.** People sometimes stereotype those with disabilities, assuming their quality of life (QOL) is poor or that they are unhealthy because of their impairments.
- **Stigma, prejudice, and discrimination.** Within society, these attitudes may come from people's ideas related to disability—people may see disability as a personal tragedy, as something that needs to be cured or prevented, as a punishment for wrongdoing, or as an indication of the lack of ability to behave as expected in society.

Nowadays, society's understanding of disability is improving as we recognize "disability" as what occurs when a person's functional needs are not addressed in her or his physical and social environment. By not considering disability a personal deficit or shortcoming, and instead thinking of it as a social responsibility in which all people can be supported to live independent and full lives, it becomes easier to recognize and address challenges that all people—including those with disabilities—experience.

Communication Barriers

Communication barriers are experienced by people who have disabilities that affect hearing, speaking, reading, writing, and/or understanding, and who use different ways to communicate than people who do not have these disabilities. Examples of communication barriers include:

- Written health promotion messages with barriers that prevent people with vision impairments from receiving the message. These include:
  - Use of small print or no large-print versions of material
  - No braille or versions for people who use screen readers
- Auditory health messages may be inaccessible to people with hearing impairments, including:
  - Videos that do not include captioning
  - Oral communications without accompanying manual interpretation (such as, American Sign Language (ASL))
- The use of technical language, long sentences, and words with many syllables may be significant barriers to understanding for people with cognitive impairments.

Physical Barriers

Physical barriers are structural obstacles in natural or human-made environments that prevent or block mobility (moving around in the environment) or access. Examples of physical barriers include:

- Steps and curbs that block a person with mobility impairment from entering a building or using a sidewalk
- Mammography equipment that requires a woman with mobility impairment to stand
- Absence of a weight scale that accommodates wheelchairs or others who have difficulty stepping up

Policy Barriers

Policy barriers are frequently related to a lack of awareness or enforcement of existing laws and regulations that require programs and activities be accessible to people with disabilities. Examples of policy barriers include:

- Denying qualified individuals with disabilities the opportunity to participate in or benefit from federally funded programs, services, or other benefits
- Denying individuals with disabilities access to programs, services, benefits, or opportunities to participate as a result of physical barriers
- Denying reasonable accommodations to qualified individuals with disabilities, so they can perform the essential functions of the job for which they have applied or have been hired to perform

Programmatic Barriers

Programmatic barriers limit the effective delivery of a public-health or healthcare program for people with different types of impairments. Examples of programmatic barriers include:

- Inconvenient scheduling
- Lack of accessible equipment (such as mammography screening equipment)
- Insufficient time set aside for medical examination and procedures
- Little or no communication with patients or participants
- Provider's attitudes, knowledge, and understanding of people with disabilities

Social Barriers

Social barriers are related to the conditions in which people are born, grow, live, learn, work, and age—or social determinants of health—that can contribute to decreased functioning among people with disabilities. Here are examples of social barriers:

- People with disabilities are far less likely to be employed. In 2017, 35.5 percent of people with disabilities, ages 18 to 64 years, were employed, while 76.5 percent of people without disabilities were employed, about double that of people with disabilities.
- Adults aged 18 years and older with disabilities are less likely to have completed high school compared to their peers without disabilities (22.3 % compared to 10.1%).
- People with disabilities are more likely to have income of less than $15,000 compared to people without disabilities (22.3% compared to 7.3%).
- Children with disabilities are almost four times more likely to experience violence than children without disabilities.

Transportation Barriers

Transportation barriers are due to a lack of adequate transportation that interferes with a person's ability to be independent and to function in society. Examples of transportation barriers include:
- Lack of access to accessible or convenient transportation for people who are not able to drive because of vision or cognitive impairments
- Public transportation may be unavailable or at inconvenient distances or locations

CHAPTER 64
SOCIAL SKILLS, FRIENDS, AND DATING

About This Chapter: "Social Skills, Friends, and Dating," © 2017 Omnigraphics. Reviewed July 2020.

Not all of the effects of learning disabilities (LDs) are related to academic success. In addition to school-related issues, teens with LD often experience difficulties with making friends and forming romantic relationships. Although the social skills involved in these personal interactions come naturally to many people, you may need help or training to develop these skills if you have learning or attention issues. This sort of training can provide important benefits in the classroom and contribute to successful relationships later in life.

Some learning and attention issues can have a direct impact on your social skills and lead to social isolation or rejection. If you struggle with visual or auditory perception, for instance, you may not notice or understand facial expressions, vocal inflection, or other social "cues" as easily as your peers. As a result, you may have trouble gauging and responding to the moods of people you interact with. If you have spatial awareness issues, you may struggle with the concept of personal space. You may stand closer to other people than they are comfortable with while talking to them. Some teens with attention issues may behave impulsively or disruptively without thinking through all the potential consequences of their actions. Others may have trouble setting realistic goals, being well-organized, and staying on task. These issues can create frustration for their classmates and negatively affect social relationships.

Building Social Skills
Fortunately, parents and teachers can help teens with LD learn strategies to deal with social situations. Special social skills training is also available through school- or community-based counseling services. By working to improve your social skills, you will be able to interact more positively with your peers, which may also help improve your academic performance.

Some of the techniques and strategies for teaching social skills include the following:

- **Role-playing**—Role-playing enables you to learn about and practice using social conventions in a safe environment. Taking turns with an adult, you can think up situations that require good social skills and model appropriate responses. This technique can also be useful in helping you recognize facial expressions and interpret vocal tone. The adult can model certain moods or expressions and have you guess what they are. Another way to observe nonverbal behavior is by watching television with the sound muted and discussing what each character is trying to convey with their body language.

- **Body awareness**—Teens with LD sometimes struggle with a lack of awareness of their body position. One strategy for addressing this issue is to perform everyday physical activities such as sitting down, standing up, climbing stairs, or eating while a parent records you with a video camera. Watching yourself on video can help you increase awareness of your physical positioning and reduce movements that may appear socially awkward.

- **Receiving information**—Teens with LD often need to receive information in specific ways in order to remember or process it effectively. Asking for help in receiving information is an important social skill that should be developed in school. You can work with your teachers to learn polite methods of requesting information or accommodations. Instead of saying "I don't get it," for instance, the teacher might encourage you to say, "Could you please explain the directions to me again so I can be sure I understand?"

- **Organizational skills**—Disorganization can make life more complicated for anyone. For teens with LD, however, it can lead to visual distraction, time-consuming searches, and frustrating delays. Learning to organize things is a valuable skill that can lead to improvements in many other areas. You can work with your parents and teachers to develop better organizational skills and strategies. For example, you might devise a system for putting everything you need for school in a specific place the night before to save time in the morning.

- **Conversation skills**—It can be difficult for some teens with LD to understand the hidden rules of conversation. Without coping strategies, they may tend to dominate conversations or avoid participating completely. Social skills training can help you develop strategies for improving your conversational skills, such as making eye contact, nodding to show that you are listening, or looking puzzled if you need someone to explain something further. It may also be helpful to memorize a basic response to common questions, like "what do you do?" to make small talk easier.

> **Did You Know...**
> Studies have shown that 70 percent of students with LD report having "major difficulty" relating to their peers, compared to only 15 percent of nondisabled students.

Making Friends

The academic and social challenges facing teens with LD can make it difficult to form friendships. The skills required in making and keeping friends—such as talking, listening, sharing, and understanding—may not always come naturally to you. You may feel as if you do not fit in with your classmates, and you may wish that you were included in more group activities. Difficulty in making friends can impact your confidence and self-esteem and prevent you from getting involved in new things. In addition, research has shown that teens without close friends are more likely to drop out of school, abuse substances, and get in trouble with the law.

Fortunately, talking about your feelings with your parents can help you feel better about yourself. The strategies listed above can help you strengthen your social and communication skills, which can give you more confidence in connecting with other teens. It may also be helpful to ask your teachers to observe your interactions with classmates and provide feedback about your strengths and weaknesses. You can analyze various social interactions to determine what went well and identify areas to work on for next time. Finally, it is important to note that many friendships among teens are built upon shared interests in music, sports, computers, or other activities. You may be more likely to form lasting friendships by joining teams, clubs, or groups made up of people who share your interests.

Dating

For teens with LD who have trouble with ordinary social interactions, dating can be very challenging. The social cues involved in romantic relationships are even more confusing than those involved in platonic friendship. To develop the skills needed to have successful relationships, experts offer the following suggestions:

- **Find good role models**—Happy couples can shed light on the secrets to forming solid, lasting relationships. Identify positive relationship role models among your family or friends and watch how they speak to and treat each other.
- **Observe dating interactions**—There are many other examples of romantic social interaction—both positive and negative—on television, in the movies, at the mall, or in the hallways at school. You can observe these interactions for instructive lessons about human behavior, such as making eye contact, appropriate touching, and flirting.

- **Take failure in stride**—The difficult truth is that most teenage romantic relationships are temporary. As a result, it can be helpful to view dating experiences as opportunities for self-reflection, learning, and improvement. Think about the positive and negative aspects of the interaction and use that information on your next date.

References

1. Brown, Dale S. "Finding Friends and Persuading People: Teaching the Skills of Social Interaction," LD Online, September–October 1987.
2. Hayes, Marnell L. "Social Skills: The Bottom Line for Adult LD Success," LD Online, 2015.
3. "How Learning and Attention Issues Can Cause Trouble with Making Friends," Understood.org, 2016.
4. Lavoie, Rick. "Helping the Socially Isolated Child Make Friends." LD Online, 2015.
5. Rosen, Peg. "At a Glance: Dating Hurdles for Teens with Learning and Attention Issues," Understood.org, 2016.
6. Sacks, Melinda. "The Challenges of Romance for Teens with LD," GreatSchools, March 10, 2010.
7. "Social Skills and Learning Disabilities," Learning Disabilities Association of America (LDA), 2017.

CHAPTER 65
STOPPING BULLIES

About This Chapter: This chapter includes text excerpted from "Bullying and Youth with Disabilities and Special Health Needs," StopBullying.gov, U.S. Department of Health and Human Services (HHS), July 23, 2018.

Children with disabilities—such as physical, developmental, intellectual, emotional, and sensory disabilities—are at an increased risk of being bullied. Any number of factors— physical vulnerability, social skill challenges, or intolerant environments—may increase the risk. Research suggests that some children with disabilities may bully others as well.

Kids with special health needs, such as epilepsy or food allergies, also may be at higher risk of being bullied. Bullying can include making fun of kids because of their allergies or exposing them to the things they are allergic to. In these cases, bullying is not just serious, it can mean life or death.

Creating a Safe Environment for Youth with Disabilities

Special considerations are needed when addressing bullying in youth with disabilities. There are resources to help kids with disabilities who are bullied or who bully others. Youth with disabilities often have Individualized Education Programs (IEPs) or Section 504 plans that can be useful in crafting specialized approaches for preventing and responding to bullying. These plans can provide additional services that may be necessary. Additionally, civil rights laws protect students with disabilities against harassment.

Creating a Safe Environment for Youth with Special Health Needs

Youth with special health needs—such as diabetes requiring insulin regulation, food allergies, or youth with epilepsy—may require accommodations at school. In these cases, they do not require an Individualized Education Program or Section 504 plan. However, schools can protect students with special health needs from bullying and related dangers. If a child with special health needs has a medical reaction, teachers should address the medical situation first before responding to the bullying. Educating kids and teachers about students' special health needs and the dangers associated with certain actions and exposures can help keep kids safe.

Federal Civil Rights Laws and Youth with Disabilities

When bullying is directed at a child because of her or his established disability and it creates a hostile environment at school, bullying behavior may cross the line and become "disability harassment." Under Section 504 of the Rehabilitation Act of 1973 and Title II of the Americans with Disabilities Act of 1990, the school must address the harassment.

Bullying Prevention for Children with Special Healthcare Needs

Having special healthcare needs due to neurological, developmental, physical, and mental-health conditions can add to the challenges children and young people face as they learn to navigate social situations in school and in life. While bullying and cyberbullying is an unfortunate reality for many young people, children with special healthcare needs are at greater risk for being targeted by their peers.

One reason children and young adults with special healthcare needs might be at higher risk for bullying is lack of peer support. Having friends who are respected by peers can prevent and protect against bullying. Ninety-five percent of 6- to 21-year-old students with disabilities were served in public schools in 2013. However, children with special healthcare needs may have difficulty getting around the school, trouble communicating and navigating social interactions, or may show signs of vulnerability and emotional distress. These challenges can make them be perceived as different, and increase their risk of aggression from peers.

Young people with special needs may benefit from, both individualized and class-wide approaches to address the specific effects of their condition and prevent them from becoming the target or perpetrator of bullying. Teachers, school staff, and other students need to understand the specific impairments of a child's health condition, so that they can develop strategies and supports to help them participate and succeed in class and with their peers.

Potential Perceived Differences

Children and youth with special needs are impacted by their conditions in a variety of ways. Every child is unique, and so are the ways that their health condition affects them. Some impairments, such as brain injuries or neurological conditions, can impact a child's understanding of social interactions and they may not even know when they are being bullied. Here are a few ways that disabilities may affect children:

- Children and youth with cerebral palsy, spina bifida, or other neurological or physical conditions can struggle with physical coordination and speech.
- Brain injuries can impair speech, movement, comprehension, and cognitive abilities or any combination of these. A child or youth with a

brain injury may have trouble with body movements, or speaking in a way that others can understand. It could take them longer to understand what is being said or to respond.

- Children and young people with autism spectrum disorder (ASD), attention deficit hyperactivity disorder (ADHD), and Tourette syndrome may have difficulties with social interactions, sensitivities, impulsivity, and self-regulating their behavior or effectively communicating.
- A child or young person who experiences anxiety or depression or who has a mental-health condition may be withdrawn, quiet, fearful, anxious, or vulnerable. They may exhibit intense social awkwardness or have difficulty speaking.
- Children who have epilepsy or behavioral disorders may exhibit erratic or unusual behavior that makes them stand out among their peers.

Supporting Special Needs and Preventing Bullying at School

Strategies to address student's special needs at school can also help to prevent bullying and have positive outcomes for all students, especially tactics that use a team approach, foster peer relationships, and help students develop empathy. Some strategies include:

- Engaging students in developing high-interest activities in which everyone has a role to play in designing, executing, or participating in the activity
- Providing general up-front information to peers about the kinds of support children with special needs require, and have adults facilitate peer support
- Creating a buddy system for children with special needs
- Involving students in adaptive strategies in the classroom so that they participate in assisting and understanding the needs of others
- Conducting team-based learning activities and rotate student groupings
- Implementing social-emotional learning activities
- Rewarding positive, helpful, inclusive behavior

Peer Support Makes a Difference

Here are a few examples of innovative strategies used by schools to promote peer-to-peer learning, foster relationships, and prevent bullying:

- One high school created a weekly lunch program where student's with and without special healthcare needs sat and ate lunch together. Several senior students led the group, and invited their friends to join. All kinds of students participated. The students got to know each other through question and answer periods and discussions over lunch. They discovered things they had in common and formed friendships. A group of them went to the prom together.

- Youth at one school held a wheelchair soccer night. Students with special healthcare needs that used wheelchairs coached their peers in how to use and navigate the wheelchairs to play. The students helped another peer who used a wheelchair who was interested in photography by mounting a digital camera on her or his chair so she or he could be the game photographer.
- Another school created a club rule that required clubs to rotate leadership responsibilities in club meetings so that every member had a chance to run the group. This allowed students with special healthcare needs to take on leadership roles.

Peer support is an important protective factor against bullying. By working together, teachers, parents, and students can develop peer education, team-building, and leadership activities that foster friendships, build empathy, and prevent bullying to make schools safer and inclusive for all students, including children with special healthcare needs.

CHAPTER 66
SIBLINGS WITH LEARNING DISABILITIES

About This Chapter: "Siblings with Learning Disabilities," © 2020 Omnigraphics. Reviewed July 2020.

The recognition and sensitivity towards individuals with learning disabilities (LDs) have created a less restrictive and more accessible environment in educational as well as industrial institutions. Families of individuals with LD have also gained attention and various services are being offered for their education and support. However, the siblings of those with learning disabilities have been neglected as part of the effort to attend to disability issues.

Problems Faced by Siblings of Teens with Learning Disabilities
There are several difficulties faced as a member of a "specially blended family" (a family that includes members with learning disabilities and members without). Siblings of children with disabilities are at a higher risk of developing emotional issues, anxiety, and stress. They also foster an "internalizing" issue, which maybe an attempt by these siblings to hide their troubles. Other such difficulties include peer problems and a lack of commitment in extracurricular and academic activities.

Overly Responsible and Independent
In some cases, siblings experience "parentification," where they are expected to have many responsibilities for themselves and their sibling, leading them to develop duties similar to those of a parent and neglecting their own needs. This may seem favorable to parents but may lead to emotional distress in the adolescent. During teenage years, siblings often feel an increased burden to care for their siblings and parents may rely on teens to help more with household chores.

If certain responsibilities, such as babysitting, are made a choice, it helps teens feel that they have control over how much they can help out. For instance, "It'd be nice if you can watch your brother, but its okay if you want to hang out with friends." It is also important to lower expectations with regards to chores, schoolwork, or extracurricular activities since teenagers often tend to feel the burden to be perfect to make sure their parents do not have to worry about them.

Provoking a Reaction

Sibling issues may also arise from direct interactions between children, such as when a child with LD or attention deficit hyperactivity disorder (ADHD) may provoke their siblings. For instance, the child with LD may be impulsive, moody, or disorganized at home, and the other sibling may respond by being confrontational or distant. It is equally important to recognize that the child with LD may resent how easy it is for her/his sibling to finish assignments, manage time, make friends, excel in extracurricular activities, and get compliments from parents.

Feeling Neglected and Uninformed

Focusing on the child with LD may take away all the attention desired by the other sibling. Spending time on medical and therapy appointments for the child with the disability limits the amount of time parents can spend with the other children, resulting in their feeling neglected. Also, parents may spend a great deal of emotional energy on the child with the disability, leaving little emotional energy to support the sibling.

Teens may also have questions about the sibling with LD similar to parents but have little information or resources available. Parents may wish to keep siblings away from the treatment environment, leaving them clueless about what is going on with their sibling. With little or no information, they may develop their own ideas about what is happening, which is often much worse than the reality. It is necessary for parents to talk with their affected children and adolescents about learning disabilities.

Sibling Abuse

A certain level of sibling rivalry can be expected, even when one child has a learning disability. But sometimes the rivalry turns into abuse, and if there is a possibility that the sibling relationship has become abusive, parents should seek professional help. A few common signs of sibling abuse are:

- Siblings avoiding each other
- Changes in behavior, sleep patterns, eating habits, or having nightmares
- Acting out abuse while playing
- Acting in a sexually inappropriate way
- Increased violence between siblings
- The siblings' roles are rigid: one is always the offender, and the other is the victim

Experiencing Mixed Emotions

Siblings may experience a range of emotions about their situation. They may feel guilt thinking that they caused the disability of their sibling, or they may feel guilty about why the disability did not affect them. Feelings such as resentment, anger, or jealousy towards their sibling may also be experienced, considering the attention and resources spent on their sibling. Another familiar feeling is being embarrassed as a result of their sibling's disability. This can cause them to disassociate from the sibling or claim to be an only child and not invite friends over, to avoid answering questions about their sibling with LD.

Impact on Adult Lives

Teens are at a phase in life where they struggle with their independence from parents. And a teen who has a sibling with special needs may also be concerned with the idea of being apart from that sibling. It is normal and healthy for a teenager to prefer more independence and experience the world, and it should be encouraged within safe limits. As teens near adulthood, they might be troubled about the future, and wonder who is going to take care of the sibling once they have moved out. However, helping with caring for her or his sibling should depend based on the level of comfort of the individual. It is also essential to have a plan ready for when changes come that will benefit all members of the family.

Beyond the difficulties associated with having a sibling with an LD, this circumstance may also develop certain positive attributes in a teen. This includes self-control, empathy, cooperation, tolerance, compassion, maturity, and responsibility. They may also develop a sense of loyalty and a protective attitude toward their sibling. About 76 percent of adolescents understand students with a disability better due to their experience with a dyslexic sibling. In some cases, teens use a person's attitude towards special needs as a test for screening friends, and their involvement with the sibling with LD may even result in them choosing future occupations in supporting professions.

References

1. "How Learning Disabilities Affect a Child's Siblings," GreatSchools, March 14, 2016.
2. Grossman, Judy. "The Impact of LD on Siblings," Smart Kids with Learning Disabilities®, December 9, 2019.
3. Hirsch, Larissa. "Caring for Siblings of Kids with Special Needs," The Nemours Foundation/KidsHealth®, August 26, 2015.
4. Milevsky, Avidan. "Siblings of Children with Disabilities," Psychology Today, June 7, 2014.

CHAPTER 67
BECOMING A SUCCESSFUL ADULT

Most difficulties that are experienced by children with learning disabilities (LDs) continue through to adulthood. Despite similar backgrounds and LD, there are a few individuals who are able to have a successful and rewarding life by becoming productive members of society. Meanwhile, there are others who are unable to keep up emotionally, socially, or financially. Teens with learning disabilities are often considered lazy or distracted, but this is a mental disorder and should be given proper attention. Still, it is uplifting to know that there are Hollywood, business, and professional sportspeople who have overcome their learning disability to succeed in their field of expertise.

Some of the most famous celebrities such as Keanu Reeves, Tom Cruise, and Daniel Radcliffe, are known to suffer from dyslexia. Tommy Hilfiger, the fashion designer, is also dyslexic, but his condition helped him see things differently and create a unique style. Musicians including Adam Levine and Justin Timberlake suffered from attention deficit disorder (ADD), and Michael Phelps, who won 28 Olympic swimming medals, was diagnosed with attention deficit hyperactivity disorder (ADHD). A few other celebrity actors who suffered from LD include Whoopi Goldberg, Keira Knightley, Woody Harrelson, Mark Ruffalo, and Jay Leno.

Attributes of Success
Success means different things to people at various times in their life. As an adult, success primarily consists of having a good social life, self-approval, job satisfaction, mental- and physical-health, financial stability, spiritual contentment, and a purpose in life. Each of these components of success has a lesser or greater emphasis, depending upon the individual's perspective. Researchers at the Forstig Center in Pasadena, CA have conducted a 20-yearlong study to identify specific personal characteristics, behaviors, and attitudes that attribute to success in people with LD. They figured that there are six major attributing factors for success in people with LD:
- Disability self-awareness

- Proactive behavior
- Being perseverant
- Setting realistic goals
- Making use of effective support systems
- Developing strategies for emotional coping

Being Self-Aware

Successful people who have learning disabilities are usually aware of their limitations and they understand how this affects their lives. It is also important to note that these individuals possess the ability to compartmentalize their disability and they view it as a single aspect of their whole self. They recognize their talents and strengths as well as accept their limitations, but are not defined by them. For instance, an individual with math deficits but excellent writing skills might refuse to choose a career in accounting, and yet be a successful journalist.

Proactivity

Being proactive is another factor that successful adults with LD share in common. They tend to participate in community activities and play an active role in their family and social settings. It helps them demonstrate a creative self-advocacy and take initiative, whereas unsuccessful individuals play the role of a passive observer and merely respond to events. Assuming responsibility for your actions and having the ability to make decisions and act upon those decisions is another contributing factor to success. It is also necessary to have the willingness to consult with others and weigh the options when making decisions.

Ability to Persevere

Individuals with LD must show perseverance when pursuing their chosen path and not give up easily, despite the challenges they face. They should not give up on their goals and search for alternative ways to reach it, depending on the circumstances. However, it is also important to know when to quit or change their goals for a better chance at success. There may be numerous difficult situations for young adults with LD when compared to their peers. However, these are considered necessary to overcome adversity and hardships that may occur at a later point in life.

Goal Setting

Specific, yet flexible tentative goals should be set during adolescence, so that they can be altered to suit specific situations, for individuals with LD to be successful in life. Goals can comprise several areas including studies, work, relationships, spiritual, and personal development. Along with goals, a person with LD also requires specific step-by-step strategies to reach their objective. It is also important to have achievable and realistic goals, which provide a purpose in their lives. For instance, a person with severe eye–hand coordination problems and spatial relations issues cannot aim to become a pilot.

Effective Social Support Systems

An individual with LD generally receives support and assistance at a young age from family members, mentors, therapists, and teachers. Assistance provided to adolescents should be consistent to help them reach their goals and hold clear, realistic expectations of outcomes, without being critical of their choices. As they move into adulthood, this dependence is reduced and they learn to manage on their own. To become successful, persons with LD must actively seek out help, instead of passively waiting for help to arrive, and also be willing to accept help, when offered.

Emotional Coping

A learning disability often causes stress in various settings including school, home, work, and social life. Sometimes, stress can be significant enough to result in psychological problems such as depression and anxiety. At an early age, effective means of coping and reducing stress, frustration, and other such emotional aspects of LD should be developed. The following are three major components of emotional coping:

- **Being aware of stress triggers**—such as anxiety caused by reading aloud in a group
- **Recognizing when stress develops**—physical symptoms including rapid breathing
- **Access to coping strategies**—slow deep breathing mechanism can help reduce the anxiety

Other such strategies for coping with emotional stress include seeking counseling, requesting for help, periodically changing activities, expressing feelings, being assertive, and obtaining medication if required. These are a few common coping mechanisms developed by successful people with LD to regain emotional stability.

References

1. Raskind, Marshall H.; Goldberg, Roberta J. "Life Success for Students with Learning Disabilities: A Parent's Guide," LD Online, August 25, 2003.
2. "The Famous Faces of Learning Disorders," University of Utah Health, July 26, 2017.
3. "Famous People with LD and ADHD," GreatSchools, March 4, 2010.

CHAPTER 68

SOUND ADVICE: HIGH SCHOOL MUSIC TRAINING SHARPENS LANGUAGE SKILLS

About This Chapter: This chapter includes text excerpted from "Sound Advice: High School Music Training Sharpens Language Skills," National Institutes of Health (NIH), July 28, 2015. Reviewed July 2020.

When children enter the first grade, their brains are primed for learning experiences, significantly more so, in fact, than adult brains. For instance, scientists have documented that musical training during grade school produces a signature set of benefits for the brain and for behavior—benefits that can last a lifetime, whether or not people continue to play music.

Now, researchers at Northwestern University, Evanston, Illinois, have some good news for teenagers who missed out on learning to play musical instruments as young kids. Even when musical training is not started until high school, it produces meaningful changes in how the brain processes sound. And those changes have positive benefits not only for a teen's musical abilities, but also for skills related to reading and writing.

To test the influence of musical training on the teenage brain, the National Institutes of Health (NIH)-funded researchers, led by Nina Kraus, recruited 40 rising high school freshmen shortly before the school year started. As described in the journal *Proceedings of the National Academy of Sciences (NAS)*, the students—none of whom had previous musical training—attended public schools in low-income neighborhoods in the Chicago area.

Half of the students chose to enroll in a high school band class, involving two to three hours per week of group instruction in instrumental music. The other half opted for a Junior Reserve Officers' Training Corps (ROTC) program that focused on physical fitness.

The researchers tested the students' neural responses to sound and their language skills, initially before they received musical or fitness training and then again in the summer preceding their senior year. Importantly, at entry into the study, the researchers found no difference between the groups in IQ, sex, age, or maternal education, which is a reflection of socioeconomic status. They also found no difference in neural or linguistic skills.

As Kraus explains in a fascinating video slideshow, the signals that the brain's neurons fire off in response to sound look remarkably similar to the sound waves themselves. When you play those brain waves back, you can actually hear a recognizable version of whatever the person just heard, whether the music is heavy metal or Mozart!

During adolescence, researchers have found that the brain typically becomes less reliable in the way it responds to sound. (This finding probably comes as no great surprise to anyone who has ever parented or taught teenagers.) However, the new study revealed that the brains of teens who took band classes displayed a more consistent, mature response to sound than the brains of those who took ROTC fitness classes. Now that is really something, because the neural signals the researchers were measuring reflect an automatic brain response that a person cannot voluntarily control. Therefore, the results show that the brains of the students who received musical training were physically wired to process sound more efficiently than the brains of the students who received fitness training.

What is more, the band students were better than the ROTC students at picking out speech sounds in spoken words. Kraus has shown in other studies, including a NIH-funded study in very young children reported in *PLoS Biology*, that the same brain measures of sound processing predict a child's future reading skills. In other words, the brain response to sound predicts whether or not a pre-reader will struggle in literacy development. In older children, the brain response predicts if they have been diagnosed with a learning disability, suggesting a potential clinical use for the technology that Kraus and her team have developed.

Of course, none of this discounts the value of physical education. Students who took part in the ROTC fitness program surely saw benefits in other areas. Ideally, students should be exposed to both! Still, at a time when budget constraints may make it tempting to cut school music programs, this research serves as a reminder that, just as the rest of the body benefits from physical exercise, the brain has the potential to grow stronger with the right kind of mental workouts.

CHAPTER 69

INDIVIDUALS WITH DISABILITIES EDUCATION ACT

About This Chapter: "Individuals with Disabilities Education Act," © 2017 Omnigraphics. Reviewed July 2020.

The Individuals with Disabilities Education Act (IDEA) is a U.S. law enacted to ensure that children with disabilities are provided with the same "equality of opportunity, full participation, independent living, and economic self-sufficiency" as those without disabilities. In 1990, this legislation replaced the 1975 Education for All Handicapped Children Act (EHA), and since then it has been amended several times.

There are four distinct parts to IDEA. Part A describes the general provisions of the act and establishes the Office of Special Education Programs (OSEP), which is responsible for administering the law. Part B creates educational guidelines for all school-age children with disabilities. Part C covers children from birth to age three. And Part D describes programs and activities created at the federal level to support children with disabilities.

Six Principles of Individuals With Disabilities Education Act

Individuals with Disabilities Education Act sets forth six main principles, which have essentially been in place since 1975, and with which state and local school districts must comply if they are to receive federal funding:

Free Appropriate Public Education (FAPE)

Individuals with Disabilities Education Act requires that all children, regardless of severity or type of disability, receive an education without cost to their parents, other than normal costs assessed to all students, and that the educational services be appropriate to the student's "unique needs and prepare them for further education, employment, and independent living." To this end, an individualized education program (IEP) must be developed for each student, specifying her or his needs and describing the educational services that will be provided to help the student progress in the general education curriculum.

Appropriate Evaluation

This principle is in place for two reasons: first, to ensure that the student is eligible according to the IDEA definition of a disability, and second, to determine her or his particular educational needs so that an appropriate IEP can be developed. The evaluation must include relevant information from a number of sources, including parents, teachers, classroom observation, and formal testing by experts. Schools are required to provide the evaluation free of charge, and if parents disagree with the conclusions, they have the right to request an independent evaluation, also without charge. They may also get an independent evaluation at their own expense at any time.

Individualized Education Program

The Individualized Education Program (IEP) is a written, legal document developed by an IEP team made up of parents, educators, specialists, and the student, when appropriate. It must include an assessment of the student's current educational performance, measurable annual goals, short-term objectives, and an account of the student's participation in the general curriculum. It also describes the special educational services and support the student will receive and how they will help her or him meet specific goals and objectives. IDEA requires the IEP to be reviewed and revised at least annually by the IEP team, but it is a living document that may be reviewed as often as necessary throughout the year.

Least Restrictive Environment

Individuals with Disabilities Education Act requires that students with disabilities be educated alongside those without disabilities as much as possible and that those with disabilities be moved to separate classrooms or buildings only when the severity of their condition would prevent them from receiving an appropriate education otherwise. Thus, the team and the school must make every effort to provide the necessary modifications, supplementary aid, special materials, and support needed for the student to succeed in the general educational environment. If this is not possible, plans must be made for the best possible Least Restrictive Environment (LRE) for the student outside of the regular classroom.

Parent and Student Participation in Decision Making

When IDEA was reauthorized in 2014, it was amended to make it clear that parents and, whenever possible, the student are full and equal participants in the education process. As a result, state agencies and local school boards are required to include parents of students with disabilities in any group or meeting that will make decisions about their child's IEP or LRE. They are also entitled to receive timely notice of relevant meetings, request that meetings be rescheduled so they can attend, approve or refuse additional evaluations of the student, and approve the release of any information about their child.

Procedural Safeguards

Individuals with Disabilities Education Act establishes a number of safeguards to protect the rights of children with disabilities and their parents and to ensure that they have access to all the information they need to participate in the educational process. For example, the school must provide parents with an annual written parental rights notice containing information about the special education process, procedural safeguards, and the rights of students and parents under the law. Parents also have the right to receive written notice prior to any evaluation or educational placement of their child, inspect and obtain copies of the student's records, and place an explanatory statement or correction in the record if they choose to do so. When parents disagree with any decisions related to their child, they have the right to request mediation by an impartial third party. If the disagreement is not resolved, they can ask for a due-process hearing at the state level and, further, appeal the decision in state or federal court.

References

1. Heward, W.L. "Six Major Principles of IDEA," Education.com, July 19, 2013.
2. Lee, Andrew M.I., J.D. "How IDEA Protects You and Your Child," Understood. org, n.d.
3. Saleh, Matthew, J.D., M.S. "Your Child's Rights: 6 Principles of IDEA," Smart Kids with Learning Disabilities, n.d.
4. "Six Principles of IDEA: The Individuals with Disabilities Education Act," ASK Resource Center, 2013.
5. "6 Principles of IDEA," Parents Reaching Out, n.d.

CHAPTER 70
YOUR LEGAL DISABILITY RIGHTS

About This Chapter: This chapter includes text excerpted from "Your Legal Disability Rights," USA.gov, June 3, 2020.

Discrimination and Harassment at Your Job

The Equal Employment Opportunity Commission (EEOC) (www.eeoc.gov) enforces federal laws prohibiting employment discrimination. These laws protect employees and job applicants against:

- Discrimination, harassment, and unfair treatment in the workplace by anyone because of:
  - Race
  - Color
  - Religion
  - Sex (including gender identity, transgender status, and sexual orientation)
  - Pregnancy
  - National origin
  - Age (40 or older)
  - Disability
  - Genetic information
- Being denied reasonable workplace accommodations for disability or religious beliefs
- Retaliation because they:
  - Complained about job discrimination
  - Helped with an investigation or lawsuit

Traveling with a Disability

People with disabilities have legal protection from discrimination while travelling. The Americans with Disabilities Act (ADA) gives guidelines for accessibility and special accommodations.

Voter Accessibility Laws

Voter accessibility laws ensure that people with disabilities or language barriers are able to vote.

If you know you will need accommodations on Election Day, contact your state or local election office to find out what to expect at your polling place (www.usa.gov/election-office).

Note: Many voters with disabilities rely on in-person voting at accessible polling places. Voters with language barriers often depend on the help of interpreters at the polls.

Changes to polling places are possible due to the coronavirus (COVID-19). These may include different locations, layouts, procedures, and availability of translators.

If you need to vote in person, check your polling place before Election Day. Find out about early voting options. And check with local election officials to learn:

- If your needs will be met at your polling station
- Other ways you may be able to vote

PART 8 | IF YOU NEED MORE HELP OR INFORMATION

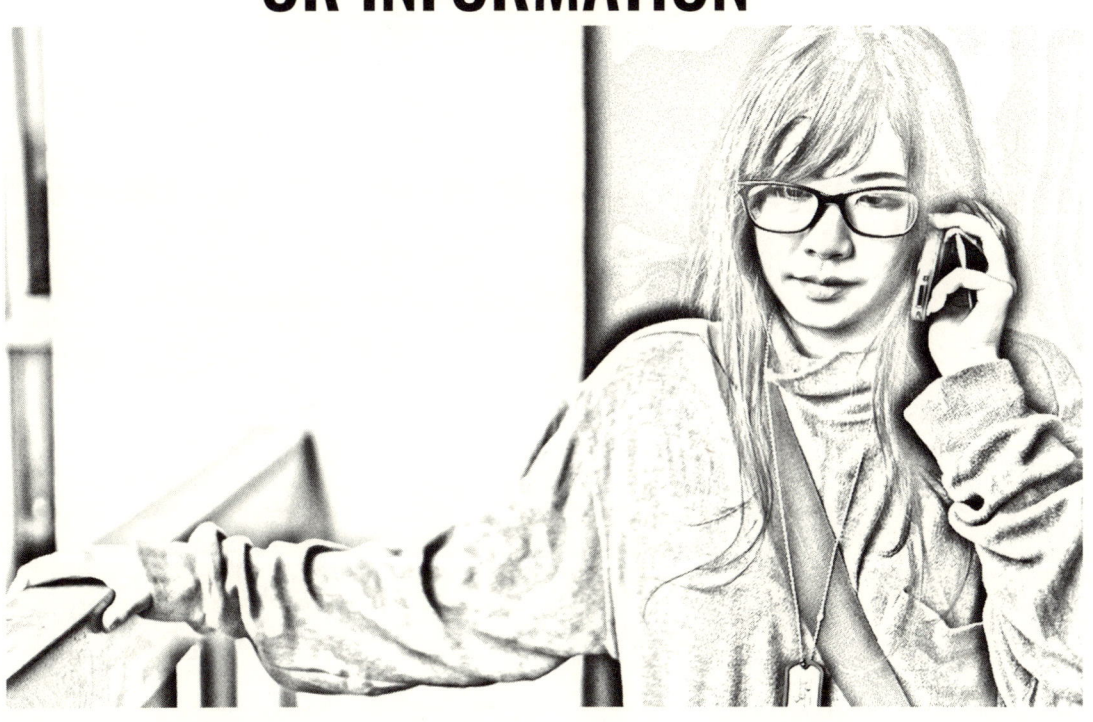

CHAPTER 71

DIRECTORY OF LEARNING DISABILITIES ORGANIZATIONS

About This Chapter: Resources in this chapter were compiled from several sources deemed reliable; all contact information was verified and updated in July 2020.

Government Agencies That Provide Information about Learning Disabilities

Centers for Disease Control and Prevention (CDC)

1600 Clifton Rd. N.E.
MS D-28
Atlanta, GA 30333
Toll-Free: 800-CDC-INFO (800-232-4636)
Toll-Free TTY: 888-232-6348
Website: www.cdc.gov
E-mail: CDC-INFO@cdc.gov

Eunice Kennedy Shriver National Institute of Child Health and Human Development (NICHD)

P.O. Box 3006
Rockville, MD 20847
Toll-Free: 800-370-2943
Toll-Free TTY: 888-320-6942
Toll-Free Fax: 866-760-5947
Website: www.nichd.nih.gov
E-mail: NICHDInformationResourceCenter@mail.nih.gov

Genetic and Rare Diseases Information Center (GARD)

P.O. Box 8126
Gaithersburg, MD 20898-8126
Toll-Free: 888-205-2311
Website: rarediseases.info.nih.gov

Genetics Home Reference (GHR)

8600 Rockville Pike
Bethesda, MD 20894
Website: ghr.nlm.nih.gov

National Institute of Neurological Disorders and Stroke (NINDS)

P.O. Box 5801
Bethesda, MD 20824
Toll-Free: 800-352-9424
Website: www.ninds.nih.gov

National Institute of Mental Health (NIMH)

6001 Executive Blvd.
Rm. 6200, MSC 9663
Bethesda, MD 20892-9663
Toll-Free: 866-615-6464
Toll-Free TTY: 866-415-8051
TTY: 301-443-8431
Fax: 301-443-4279
Website: www.nimh.nih.gov/site-info
E-mail: nimhinfo@nih.gov

National Institute on Deafness and Other Communication Disorders (NIDCD)

National Institutes of Health (NIH)
31 Center Dr.
MSC 2320
Bethesda, MD 20892-2320
Toll-Free: 800-241-1044
Toll-Free TTY: 800-241-1055
Website: www.nidcd.nih.gov
E-mail: nidcdinfo@nidcd.nih.gov

National Institutes of Health (NIH)

9000 Rockville Pike
Bethesda, MD 20892
Phone: 301-496-4000
TTY: 301-402-9612
Website: www.nih.gov

National Library Service for the Blind and Print Disabled (NLS)

Library of Congress (LOC)
1291 Taylor St. N.W.
Washington, DC 20542
Toll-Free: 800-424-8567
Phone: 202-707-5100
TDD: 202-707-0744
Fax: 202-707-0712
Website: www.loc.gov/nls
E-mail: nls@loc.gov

U.S. Department of Education (ED)

400 Maryland Ave. S.W.
Washington, DC 20202
Toll-Free: 800-USA-LEARN (800-872-5327)
Website: www.ed.gov

U.S. Department of Health and Human Services (HHS)

200 Independence Ave. S.W.
Washington, DC 20201
Toll-Free: 877-696-6775
Website: www.hhs.gov

USA.gov

Toll-Free: 844-USA-GOV1 (844-872-4681)
Website: www.usa.gov

Youth.gov

Toll-Free: 877-231-7843
Website: www.youth.gov
E-mail: youthgov@air.org

Private Agencies That Provide Information about Learning Disabilities

American Speech-Language-Hearing Association (ASHA)

2200 Research Blvd.
Rockville, MD 20850-3289
Toll-Free: 800-638-8255
Phone: 301-296-5700
TTY: 301-296-5650
Fax: 301-296-8580
Website: www.asha.org
E-mail: nsslha@asha.org

Autism Society

6110 Executive Blvd.
Ste. 305
Rockville, MD 20852
Toll-Free: 800-328-8476
Website: www.autism-society.org
E-mail: info@autism-society.org

Center for Parent Information and Resources (CPIR)

35 Halsey St.
Fourth Fl.
Newark, NJ 07102
Phone: 973-642-8100
Website: www.parentcenterhub.org

Charles and Helen Schwab Foundation

201 Mission St.
Ste. 1950
San Francisco, CA 94105
Phone: 415-795-4920
Fax: 415-795-4921
Website: www.schwabfoundation.org
E-mail: info@schwabfoundation.org

Childhood Education International

1875 Connecticut Ave. N.W.
10th Fl.
Washington, DC 20009
Toll-Free: 800-423-3563
Phone: 202-372-9986
Website: ceinternational.io

Children and Adults with Attention-Deficit/Hyperactivity Disorder (CHADD)

4221 Forbes Blvd.
Ste. 270
Lanham, MD 20706
Toll-Free: 866-200-8098
Phone: 301-306-7070
Fax: 301-306-7090
Website: www.chadd.org
E-mail: customer_service@chadd.org

Council for Exceptional Children (CEC)

3100 Clarendon Blvd.
Ste. 600
Arlington, VA 22201-5332
Toll-Free: 888-232-7733
Website: www.cec.sped.org
E-mail: service@cec.sped.org

Council for Learning Disabilities (CLD)

11184 Antioch Rd.
P.O. Box 405
Overland Park, KS 66210
Phone: 913-491-1011
Fax: 913-491-1011
Website: www.council-for-learning-disabilities.org

Dyspraxia Foundation USA

704 Juneway Ave.
Deerfield, IL 60015
Phone: 847-947-2772
Website: www.dyspraxiausa.org

HEATH Resource Center at the National Youth Transitions Center

The George Washington University (GWU)
2134 G St. N.W.
Washington, DC 20052-0001
Website: www.heath.gwu.edu
E-mail: askheath@gwu.edu

International Dyslexia Association (IDA)

40 York Rd.
Fourth Fl.
Baltimore, MD 21204
Phone: 410-296-0232
Fax: 410-321-5069
Website: dyslexiaida.org
E-mail: info@dyslexiaida.org

Kaufman Children's Center (KCC)

6625 Daly Rd.
West Bloomfield, MI 48322
Phone: 248-737-3430
Fax: 248-737-3433
Website: www.kidspeech.com
E-mail: info@kidspeech.com

Learning Ally: Recording for the Blind and Dyslexic (RFB&D)

20 Roszel Rd.
Princeton, NJ 08540
Toll-Free: 800-221-4792
Website: www.learningally.org
E-mail: custserv@learningally.org

Learning Disabilities Association of America (LDA)

461 Cochran Rd.
Ste. 245
Pittsburgh, PA 15228
Phone: 412-341-1515
Fax: 412-344-0224
Website: ldaamerica.org
E-mail: info@LDAAmerica.org

Learning Disabilities Association of Canada (LDAC)

20 - 2420 Bank St.
Ottawa, ON K1V 8S1
Canada
Phone: 613-238-5721
Website: www.ldac-acta.ca
E-mail: info@ldac-acta.ca

Learning Disabilities Association of Newfoundland and Labrador (LDANL)

66 Kenmount Rd.
Ste. 301
St. John's, NL A1B 3V7
Canada
Phone: 709-753-1445
Fax: 709-753-4747
Website: ldanl.ca
E-mail: info@ldanl.ca

Learning Disabilities Worldwide, Inc. (LDW)

179 Bear Hill Rd.
Ste. 104
Waltham, MA 02451
Fax: 978-897-5355
Website: www.ldworldwide.org
E-mail: help@ldworldwide.org

National Aphasia Association (NAA)

P.O. Box 87
Scarsdale, NY 10583
Website: www.aphasia.org
E-mail: naa@aphasia.org

National Association of Special Education Teachers (NASET)

1250 Connecticut Ave. N.W.
Ste. 200
Washington, DC 20036
Toll-Free: 800-754-4421
Website: www.naset.org
E-mail: contactus@naset.org

National Center for Learning Disabilities (NCLD)

P.O. Box 34056
Washington, DC 20043
Website: www.ncld.org

Smart Kids with Learning Disabilities®

38 Kings Hwy. N.
Westport, CT 06880
Website: www.smartkidswithld.org
E-mail: Info@SmartKidswithLD.org

INDEX

INDEX

Page numbers that appear in *Italics* refer to tables or illustrations. Page numbers that have a small 'n' after the page number refer to citation information shown as Notes. Page numbers that appear in **Bold** refer to information contained in boxes within the chapters.

asthma
    47,XYY syndrome 109
    learning disabilities statistics 38
    Tourette syndrome (TS) 167
AT *see* assistive technology
ataxia, cerebral palsy (CP) 127
athetoid, cerebral palsy (CP) 132
attention deficit disorder (ADD)
    becoming successful adult 305
    learning disabilities **7**, 236
    pediatric sleep-disordered breathing 186
attention deficit hyperactivity disorder (ADHD)
    bullying 299
    defined 35
    fetal alcohol spectrum disorders (FASDs) 87
    47,XYY syndrome 109
    learning disabilities **7**
    overview 49–55
    Smith-Kingsmore syndrome 115
    Tourette syndrome (TS) 162
    work opportunities 235
"Attention Deficit Hyperactivity Disorder"
    (NIMH) 49n
attitudinal barriers, defined 290
auditory brainstem response (ABR), full hearing
    test 175
auditory training, cued speech 180
Autism Society, contact 322
autism spectrum disorder (ASD)
    bullying 299
    developmental disabilities 36
    47,XYY syndrome 109
    overview 143–6
    Tourette syndrome (TS) 165
"Autism Spectrum Disorder: Communication
    Problems in Children" (NIDCD) 143n
"Autism Spectrum Disorder in Teenagers and
    Adults" (CDC) 143n
auxiliary aids and services
    assistive technology 275
    postsecondary education 202
"Auxiliary Aids and Services for Postsecondary
    Students with Disabilities" (ED) 275n

B

barriers
    disabilities 289, 316
    Social Security 241
"Basics about FASDs" (CDC) 85n

"Becoming a Successful Adult"
    (Omnigraphics) 305n
behavior problem
    Aarskog-Scott syndrome 113
    fetal alcohol spectrum disorders (FASDs) 87
    Tourette syndrome (TS) 166
behavioral therapy
    attention deficit hyperactivity disorder
        (ADHD) 53
    47,XYY syndrome 111
    Tourette syndrome (TS) 163
    see also psychotherapy
Benefits Planning Query (BPQY), defined 239
bipolar affective disorder *see* bipolar disorder
bipolar disorder, overview 121–6
"Bipolar Disorder and Learning Disorders"
    (NIMH) 121n
bipolar mood disorder *see* bipolar disorder
birth defects, fetal alcohol spectrum disorders
    (FASDs) 86
blood pressure
    attention deficit hyperactivity disorder
        (ADHD) 52
    cerebral palsy (CP) 130
    childhood cancer 147
    pediatric sleep-disordered breathing 185
blood test
    bipolar disorder 124
    fetal alcohol spectrum disorders (FASDs) 87
    Tourette syndrome (TS) 161
body language *see* natural gestures
bone fractures, Klinefelter syndrome 96
braces, cerebral palsy (CP) 132
brain
    bullying 298
    cerebral palsy (CP) 127
    childhood cancer 147
    Gerstmann syndrome 75
    language skills 309
    learning disabilities research 45
    pediatric sleep-disordered breathing 185
    public-health issue 15
    Smith-Kingsmore syndrome 115
    Tourette syndrome (TS) 167
brain development, public-health issue 15
brain function, drug abuse 153
brain imaging technology, learning disabilities
    research 45
brain injury
    bullying 299

job, *continued*
  mentoring 250
  policy barriers 291
  transition plan 215
  work-based experience **196**
job accommodations
  employees with LD 236
  see also Job Accommodation Network (JAN);
    workplace accommodations
Job Accommodation Network (JAN),
  described 243
job shadowing
  mentoring 218
  work-based experience **196**
  work-based learning 250
juvenile justice, transition planning 213

K

Kaufman Children's Center (KCC), contact 324
kernicterus, jaundice 36
Klinefelter syndrome, overview 95–104
"Klinefelter Syndrome (KS): Condition
  Information" (NICHD) 95n
K-12 public schools, service-learning 269
kyphosis, co-occurring conditions of CP 133

L

language and speech disorders,
  overview 169–72
language delay
  developmental disorder 67
  fetal alcohol spectrum disorders (FASDs) 86
language development
  autism 144
  Klinefelter syndrome (KS) 101
language impairments
  special education services 193
  statistics 38
  see also specific language impairment (SLI)
late effects, cancer survivors 147
"Late Effects of Treatment for Childhood Cancer
  (PDQ®)—Patient Version" (NCI) 147n
LDA *see* Learning Disabilities Association of
  America
LDAC *see* Learning Disabilities Association of
  Canada
LDANL *see* Learning Disabilities Association of
  Newfoundland and Labrador

lead poisoning
  overview 155–7
  statistics 38
leadership
  career-specific work skills 217
  High School/High Tech (HS/HT) program **196**
  peer support 300
  student learning 274
Learning Ally: Recording for the Blind and
  Dyslexic (RFB&D), contact 324
learning assessments, students with LD 262
learning difficulties
  bipolar disorder **123**
  co-occurring conditions of CP 134
  dyscalculia **59**
  Klinefelter syndrome 98
  students with LD 261
Learning Disabilities Association of America
  (LDA), contact 324
Learning Disabilities Association of Canada
  (LDAC), contact 324
Learning Disabilities Association of
  Newfoundland and Labrador (LDANL),
  contact 324
learning disabilities (LDs)
  college planning 197
  dyslexia 25
  epilepsy 139
  gifted student 7
  lead poisoning 155
  NICHD-sponsored research 45
  reading disorder 63
  self-esteem issues 281
  sibling abuse 302
  students with LD 261
  Turner syndrome 105
  work opportunities 235
"Learning Disabilities on the Job"
  (Omnigraphics) 235n
"Learning Disabilities—What Are the
  Treatments for Learning Disabilities?"
  (NICHD) 31n
Learning Disabilities Worldwide, Inc. (LDW),
  contact 325
learning skills
  hearing loss 179
  standardized tests 27
  students with LD 261
learning strategies
  cerebral palsy (CP) 138
  self-advocacy skills 285

T